TABLE OF CON

ACKNOWLEDGEMENTS

My heart overflows with gratitude for the process of writing this book and for the many people who made it possible. Without so many, this book would have never seen the light of day.

To my coach, Courtney Seard, thank you for driving me to be my personal best and for helping me regain my health during a time I was completely lost. You've always asked the hard questions that push me outside of my comfort zone and allow me to live in my greatness. I am forever grateful for your wisdom, friendship, and guidance. You are a powerful light in this world.

My love for writing began in grad school surrounded

by the inspiring stories and poetry written by Bécquer, Neruda, Allende, Márquez, García Lorca, Esquivel and so many others. I'm so grateful for the incredible colleagues in the program and for the teachers that brought my love for literature to life. I will forever have fond memories of walking the hills of Reno with Lisa O'Neil Katzenstein while studying using our tiny notecards and dreaming of veggie burgers at Bully's. I couldn't have asked for a better partner in crime to begin my love affair with writing and literature. And there were many times during this process I channeled our adventures in Spain, Vale.

To my incredible family, especially the Dovan ladies who constantly pushed the power of my imagination to the limits and beyond. My childhood was filled with so much make-believe and fun that has helped me today become the master of metaphors. I couldn't ask for a more loving and supportive family; thank you beloved cousins! Muchas gracias Mama-Lu, Dadio, and Juju-Bee for always having my back; even when you didn't understand the path I was on, you stood alongside me.

To my amazing in-laws across the pond, I am so lucky to have married into such a wonderful and kindhearted family. Spending time on the farm with you during the holidays always brings such inspiration and pure joy.

My bad bunnies, Natasha Collins, Marisa Rodriguez, Anthea Lim Yugawa, Andrea Marchesi, Kristina Pineda, Sunanda Pejavar, and April Chu, you have made living in San Francisco one of the greatest adventures of my life.

Thank you for the endless nights of laughing so hard I fall over, for being incredible travel buddies, dance partners, and endless inspirations. My heart overflows with love for you.

To my friends who have kept me sane and supported me during this process, I stand in deep gratitude for you and your words of encouragement. There are too many to mention - most recently: Stacia Burton Rogers, Joy Aaring, Alexandra Liss, Abigayle Rosser, Oriana Branon, Michelle Gee, Barbara Hansson, Alexis Pence, Ashley Grems, Carmen Kiew, Nathaniel Bliss, Erin McElaney, Jessika Rivera, Mallory Benham and Jen Koepnick. I wouldn't be where I am today without your love and understanding.

To my ladies who I have known since childhood: Sierra Lowe, Dusty Carter, Brooke Triplett and Trisha Crisco – our combined 100 years of friendship is something I am thankful for every single day. Even miles apart and separated by time zones, you are and will forever be family.

To my talented friend and photographer, Genevieve Burruss, I cannot thank you enough for running around LA taking photos with me for this book cover. You made this awkward writer comfortable and even have a day of fun! I can't wait to travel the world with you and continue to see you wield your lens magic.

Master designer and goddess extraordinaire, Amy Barroso, thank you for bringing my visions to life and for this incredible book cover. You are an incredible teammate and visual wizard.

To all of my brave and inspiring clients and those I've had the pleasure to work with. Thank you from the bottom of my heart for putting your faith in me and in yourself. Thank you for your courage to discover a new path, for your willingness to be vulnerable and strong, and for showing up for yourselves and creating powerful change.

To my teachers and trainers at the Tad James Company who have made me the coach and person I am today – I am, mind, body, and soul, eternally grateful.

To my mentor, my inspiration and friend Marcia Wieder; you always say that *Dream* is a verb and I had no idea what you meant until I dove into my awakening with you. Thank you for challenging me in the best way possible and for unlocking my truest Dream, to live a life of inspiring others to follow their path to happiness. The name *Inspire• Magic* was born during our time together and from it has sprung my mission in life. Thank you for sharing your magic with me and continuing to share your gifts with the world. Sono grato per te.

For Oprah, Ellen DeGeneres, and incredible people like this in the world, thank you! Thank you for spreading your kindness and light and for making the world laugh and cry with joy. I can't count the number of times my sister and I spend watching Ellen for our daily dose of magic. Such a powerful message you share – Be Kind. So simple, yet has the power to change the world.

And to you dear reader, little do you know you are

already an Inspired Magician just on the brink of finding your voice, your magic and your greatness. I'm excited to be on this incredible journey with you.

With Gratitude and Love,
Michelle

NOTE FROM THE AUTHOR

My mission is to inspire you to step out of your comfort zone and into your greatness. I aim to show you a life outside of the one you thought you were destined for, and into the magic of your own creation; to touch a part of your spirit by uncovering the passion, desire, and confidence that lies just under the surface of the negative beliefs and emotions you have accrued over the years. My goal is to re-introduce you to yourself—your true self—and let that person follow your dreams to the life you have always desired. Ultimately, you only live one life, and I want you to tap into your Inspired Magic. Be a magician and create an inspired life.

PROLOGUE

Two hikers are lost and stranded in a forest at night. Having no flashlights with them, it is pitch black, but they can almost make out a faint light in the distance. It is so faint, in fact, that they believe it to be the reflection of the moon over a stream. For a while, they sit and ponder their situation, each lost in their own thoughts.

Through the inky blackness of the night, one hiker begins to focus on the shadows, the ominous shapes made by the trees, the unfamiliar cacophony of the nocturnal foragers, and the howling of the wind. This hiker is unsettled and imagines nightmarish scenarios of what may happen. She begins to see the trees as enemies, and believes the noises of the night are animals preparing to move in. She nervously wonders about leaving this site and becoming more lost. What if they fall into a stream and get wet, or worse? What if they are lost for so long that they run out of food and cannot find fresh water? What if? *What if?*

The other hiker recognizes that it is dark and acknowledges that she is lost. She chooses to focus on the faint light way off in the distance. This hiker believes that there may be people near that light; she might find people or resources, and no longer be lost. So, she steps into the darkness, one foot after the other, in the direction of the light. She beckons for the other hiker to walk with her, but this woman is petrified by the scenarios in her head, and remains behind, hoping to be found, waiting for someone to rescue her.

As the hiker, making her way towards the light, continues to walk through the forest, she notices her eyes beginning to adjust to the darkness, and the path becomes clearer. She hears raccoons and opossums bustling around her, and is comforted by nature's presence. She walks slowly but steadily through the forest, towards the light, and thinks to herself, "It does not matter how slowly I go, as long as I do not stop."

The first hiker saw darkness as the enemy, something to be feared. She allowed the darkness to petrify her; she only focused on what could go wrong. The second hiker saw darkness as that which allows light to be seen. Had she waited till morning, the visibility of that dim light would no longer be visible. She knew it was time, and so she began.

Without darkness, the faint light would have never been.

"There is no light without dark, no happiness without grief, no improvement without error, and no true love without heartbreak. Take every bump in the road as a signal for something greater to come."
– Roy Peng

A New Beginning: The Magic Starts Here

◆◆◆

"What we achieve inwardly will change outer reality."
– Plutarch

Oct 30, 2016

It is no coincidence that the last day I am in Rome, I find myself drinking a cappuccino on the terrace of the Pope, as the sun rises over the city; though this morning is slightly different, since I was awakened by a 7.1 earthquake that hit Perugia. I believe that earthquakes are Mother Nature's way of saying that we are not listening to her, and we need to wake up, especially when they happen first thing in the morning.

All I hear are the fountains and the birds. This is the same as one week ago today. How is it possible that I have already spent an entire week here? I have done more to explore Italy in one week than most tourists could do in an entire month! Though the exploration that was the most profound and meaningful to me was the exploration of my own heart and soul, as well as witnessing the interaction between my essence, and being with the breathtaking scenery around me.

We are all a bit like Rome: a city made up of ancient structures, where new-found ideas have just plopped themselves right on top of it, without clearing any of the old away. The city does a splendid job of pretending what used to live there does not exist, but all it takes is a little encouragement, and then the ancient structures reveal themselves in surprising ways. The new and the old live here together in harmony, one not quite understanding the other, but still acknowledging its existence. It is hard to say who influenced whom more when you see what resides here. Were renaissance builders inspired by ancient Roman architecture? Did the ancient Romans have their third eye open to the wonderment that could be created, if only they believed it could? One look at the Colosseum and you must wonder if God did not just drop that right out of the sky.

Before this trip, I visited my doctor's office and was told that I needed reading glasses. I had been living with a constant headache, and felt that my eyes were crossing. One day after arriving here, I could see perfectly without reading glasses. In fact, I have never seen so clearly in my entire life! My magic has been ignited here. I think about having to go back, and what that will mean for me. I do not feel the same magic back home, and I realize that it is all of my own making. Little choices that have made sense over the years are now showing their unfavorable outcomes. These were times I had decided to take the safe path, the one others approved of, the one that was what I was supposed to do. Rarely do people make decisions to please others and feel fulfilled. True fulfillment is self-initiated and self-maintained. When did I decide I could not create a life that I loved to live every single day?

There is a crossroad that we all hit, where we choose either the path of unknowing and risk, or we choose the path of the practical. Do we take the path to follow our dreams, or decide dreams do not come true for us, and follow the practical path? What makes us choose the dreamless path? Is it fear? A lack of confidence? What, exactly, tells us that we should settle? Make no mistake about it; settling is a choice. No one *makes* you do anything, although sometimes the temporary repercussions can make you choose the path more traveled—though this is not you, or at least this is not the *you* that you are becoming. After all, you picked up this book, and you have made it this far—congratulations! You have decided that it is time to create more of what you love, and get clear about how to get there.

Here is the thing: **<u>You are responsible for your change</u>**. This book is not meant to sit on your shelf with the other dozen books you may have picked up over the years. Inside the pages of this book, you will be challenged and encouraged, but the action is all on you. It is time.

In your everyday interactions, you make choices. These choices are based on your past experiences, things you have learned along the way, and how you see others making choices. Imagine that your brain is a computer, set with specific programs and wiring. As time goes on, that computer needs an update when it is not giving you the desired outcomes. Maybe the program in the past worked perfectly for you, but as your needs, environment, and desires change, your program needs to change as well.

There was a period in my life where I needed major changes. I was seeking a healthy relationship, I had health issues, and I was looking for a major career change. I hired a coach and began working with her to break down the patterns and limiting decisions that were impeding me from creating the life I wanted. Through neuro-linguistic programming (NLP), hypnotherapy, and other modalities, I was able to break through barriers that had blocked me for years.

After I saw the profound changes that working with Courtney brought to my life, I realized I needed to learn more. Now, as a trainer of NLP, and a trainer of hypnotherapy, I want to share with you what I have learned over many years. For those who are not familiar with neuro-linguistic programming, it is a set of tools and techniques, but it is so much more than that. It is an attitude and a methodology of knowing how to achieve your goals and get results.[1] *Neuro* refers to your neurology and how you organize thoughts through your five senses; *linguistic* refers to language, or how we communicate with ourselves and others; *programming* refers to how we organize our thoughts and actions to create results. In other words, learning NLP is like learning the language of your own mind!

In NLP, we have a saying: the conscious mind is the goal *setter*, and the unconscious mind is the goal *getter*.[2] Your unconscious mind will achieve for you whatever you want in life, but first you must learn how to communicate properly with your unconscious mind. When we find ourselves in a place where we are not getting the outcomes we desire, this is when we are out of rapport with our own unconscious. I will warn you, if you follow the steps in this book, you will have a positive transformation, so be prepared. Imagine what your life would be like if you were able to change that which does not serve you, and create the life you dream about. Existing within you is the ability to chase and catch what you want the most. Do you want better health? Do you want to do what you love on a daily basis? Do you want to maintain or find a thriving relationship? Do you want to build a better relationship with yourself? All of this, and more, is possible!

As you read this book, I will teach you which habits increase desired outcomes, and which habits inhibit them. I will give you processes to follow, and provide guidelines on how to use them. You will learn how to reset the way you have been doing things, and bring into light the thoughts, activities, and people who may be keeping you from living your ultimate life. And above all else, you will reignite your passion for life and find the inspiration to take the necessary action.

Never take anything at face value; do the work, put in the effort, and decide that once and for all, you have control over your outcomes, and you are the creator of your destiny. I learned this lesson many years ago and have been improving upon it ever since. In seventh grade, my social studies teacher, Mr. Kelly Dant, told me that I always have at least two choices. I was twelve years old and remember it like it was yesterday. I heard the class argue, "What if you were put into a really bad situation that was totally not your choice?" His response was eye-opening to me: he said that your reaction to what is happening around you is always your choice, even if the circumstances are not.

The lesson on choices from my social studies teacher had a profound impact on me. It can make you stop and think what brought you to those situations in the first place. Take the following analogy: A young girl goes for a walk and ends up lost. She realizes that every step she took has led her there—not just the last five steps or the first ten, but each and every step she has taken, along with every breath along the way, and every single thought that crossed her mind has led her to that very place at that very moment.

She approaches a tall, wise tree, which tells her that everything she does, thinks, and feels leads her into every situation. It was not only the steps she was paying attention to but also the ones she was not, that led her to where she found herself. In other words, the power is in your hands. Though it turns out that the path she was on was actually the one that would lead her to where she truly wanted to be; even though, while right in the middle of the journey, she may have felt as if she were not where she wanted to be. We are never truly lost; we are only in various stages of being found. What we seek are fulfillment and contentment, and it is up to you whether this is the time to follow your true calling.

What is Magic?

◆◆◆

What is Inspired Magic? My definition of magic is how we tap into the universal consciousness of infinite love and energy. It is how we create true fulfillment through self-love and connecting with the people and things that bring us optimal health and vitality. Magic is the ability to create something we desire outside of ourselves, with the power of the mind. Imagine a sunrise. Without warning nor permission, the sun begins to break up the night. If you close your eyes, you can hear her whispering promises of a better day than the one before. In that moment of every sunrise, you witness just how much magic there is in this world.

Throughout this book, I will be breaking down what increases your magic, and what decreases your magic, in three sections. Use this book as a buffet of knowledge. You do not have to do everything step by step in order to make positive changes in your life. If there is something that really speaks to you, make sure you dive in with both feet! If there is something that does not work in your life, feel free to skip it. I do urge you to think about WHY you may not want to try something outlined ahead, and ask yourself if this the area you may need the most help with. I have broken this book down into three sections.

Section one relates to the Mind. Real change starts inside and works its way out. The way you think is such a critical part of what your life becomes and how you can affect real change in it. It all starts in the mind, then works its way into words; those words turn into actions, and those actions have resulted in the life you are currently living. When you make beneficial changes on the foundational level, you allow a positive ripple effect to work its way into all areas of your life. In this section, you will learn effective goal setting, the role of limiting beliefs, and how to create a mindset that will allow you to make a big transformation in your life.

Section two relates to the Body. *Health is wealth* is a saying we have all heard, and it is true. No matter how much money you have, or how much love you have, unless you are healthy, it does not bring the same fulfillment and contentment you can have when you have optimal health. In this section you will learn how to create healthy patterns and habits that will give you more energy and less stress. There will be exercises for de-cluttering your life and clearing out negative energy. You will also learn how body language can affect your mood and energy. As you begin to live a healthier, balanced life, your energy will radiate out and attract more of what you want in other areas of your life. After all, without great health, how will you enjoy the new and improved life you are creating?

Section three relates to the Spirit. After you have learned how to improve your mind and body, it will be time to tap into the part of you that drives you forward and catches your dreams. In this section, you will discover what inspires you, and how to go beyond the Law of Attraction to take *Inspire• Action* and learn how to truly receive. You will also learn how to quiet your mind in order to hear your true inner desires. Once you do this, you will become an *Inspire• Magician.*

My mission is to remind you of who you truly are. I intend to help you let go of the baggage and the doubt, as well as the story you have told yourself over the years, which took you away from the confident person you were born to be.

Who were you before that first bully came into your life? Who were you before the first time you ever failed at anything? Who were you before that first moment you ever felt afraid? Who were you before you let emotions get the best of you, and you lashed out in anger? Let's rediscover that person; she is alive and well, inside of you. Attempts to heal these wounds may have caused you to make choices that are not in your best interest. Let's get back to loving yourself the way you are loved at a spiritual level. Let's rediscover the best version of you, so you can show up for yourself and others the way you have always wanted to.

Since completing the exercises in this book is a large part of what will help you make the changes necessary to move forward with the life you want, let us start right now. Write down one habit you want to let go, and one habit you wish to adopt, just to ease your way into doing tasks.

ONE HABIT TO ADD:

____

____

____

ONE HABIT TO SUBTRACT:

____

____

____

"As is a tale, so is life: not how long it is, but how good it is, is what matters."
– Lucius Annaeus Seneca

Inspired Thoughts

PART ONE -
MIND

"A man cannot directly choose his circumstances, but he can choose his thoughts, and so indirectly, yet surely, shape his circumstances."
– James Allen

YOUR MAGIC MIND: MANAGING MINDSETS

You may have picked up this book at a bookstore or online, or maybe a friend or family member gifted it to you. No matter how this book came into your hands, you have made the decision to read it. Great news! This means that you are ready to make some changes in your life that will allow more ease, joy, and abundance to come your way. Being open to innovative ways of thinking and being open to new behaviors are the hardest part of the journey.

Now, there may be times that you are reading through the examples and directions I give you, and you may think, well, that is not how everyone else does it. And you would be right. But as you look around, seeing people doing the same things over and over, and complaining about the same old complaints, you will quickly realize that you do not want to be just like everyone else, won't you? The only person who can stop you from achieving your goal, is you.

Every day, I see how a person's mindset affects their outcome. For example, two people of similar backgrounds and skill sets are working hard to achieve what they want. Yet often, one person achieves their goal and the other does not. There is nothing on the surface that would distinguish these two—no difference in education or development that should put one ahead of the other. Yet one does not achieve what they set out to achieve. Why does this happen?

Are you the one that gets what they set out to achieve every time, or are you the one that can taste the finish line, yet rarely crosses it? A key difference between these two people is mindset—a simple yet profound concept that separates the wishers from the doers, and the haves from the have-nots. Once you begin to develop a healthier mindset, you will begin to see opportunities you have never seen, connect with people in a new way, and take inspired actions you have never taken.

When I begin working with clients, the very first thing I tell them is this: Your unconscious mind is always eavesdropping on you. Let me repeat that again: Your unconscious mind is always eavesdropping on you. Depending on where you are entering this process, you will have varying degrees of healthy, and maybe not so healthy, self-talk. Think of all the times you have heard someone say, or have said yourself,

"If I eat that, it will go straight to my hips!" Or, "It would be impossible to do X." When we talk about the unconscious mind, we are talking about the part of you that runs in the background beyond your conscious awareness. It is the role of the unconscious mind to store and organize your memories, to run the body, and to preserve the body. It is what breathes for you at night while you are sleeping. You do not consciously remind yourself every few seconds of the day, "Okay now, body, it is time to breathe again." It is also the part of you that is going after your dreams and desires, so it is important that what your unconscious mind believes is what you want to attract into your world.

Really, the job of your unconscious is enormous! The UM (unconscious mind) is sorting through as much as 11 million bits of information every second, through our five senses. Imagine that each bit of information is a grain of sand. It may be possible to hold onto some of that sand, but 11 million grains per second, coming your way at once, would be too much to handle. How much of that 11 million bits of information, which you are receiving every single second, are you processing? The answer is only around 50–126 bits per second. This number varies, depending on the individual and the task being performed. That is not a lot compared to what is being thrown your way throughout the day.

Regardless of the scenario, you can process only a tiny fraction of information coming at you. This makes the quality of information you are paying attention to that much more important. If you were to record every thought, feeling, and word spoken, what frequency would it reflect? Are the thoughts, feelings, and words overwhelmingly positive, negative, optimistic, or pessimistic? If you are not sure, take a moment to ask yourself how you feel. Your feelings are a great barometer to calibrate your thoughts. If you are feeling bad, the thoughts going through your mind are most likely negative or pessimistic. If you find a smile on your face and a good feeling inside, you are most likely thinking good-feeling thoughts, and paying attention to the information around you that makes you feel good. In those moments, really allow yourself to feel it completely. Take it all in, notice how it feels from your head to your toes, and bathe in it for a while. Is that not really what it is all about, after all? Is not everything we seek in life so that we end up feeling happy?

It does not matter how much focus you place on your dreams, if deep down you are running an undercurrent of thoughts that sabotage your efforts. All of that negative chatter will undermine your hard work and efforts. But here is the good news: Once you realize that your unconscious mind is always listening to your every thought, your feelings, and your words, you can take control of what you choose to focus on, and change your program.

Now, I do not want you to think that you must police every thought that comes your way. That would be entirely too much work, and this book is designed to teach you the skills to bring you more joy and ease. I will explain in later chapters how to upgrade your thinking without focusing on every thought that crosses your mind. The first place to start is by removing limiting beliefs.

Inspired Thoughts

Abracadabra – Making Limiting Beliefs Disappear

So, what are the thoughts that are stopping you from achieving your goals and receiving all you want in life? They are, in large part, self-limiting beliefs. Self-limiting beliefs are mental roadblocks that stop your progress and sabotage your success. These beliefs may be a result of an experience that did not turn out how you wanted, or maybe they are beliefs that you heard as a child and have accepted as true.

A fitting example of a limiting belief that used to exist is that it was impossible to run the four-minute mile. That is to say, for many years, runners around the globe were unable to run one mile in under four minutes, despite training and coaching. Many believed it could not be done, until one day, in 1954, in Oxford, England, Roger Gilbert Bannister broke the four-minute mile, running it in 3 minutes and 59.4 seconds. After years and years of runners attempting to run a mile in under four minutes, finally, the world knew it could be done, thanks to Roger Bannister. Did it take years and years for the next person to do it? No, it was broken by Australian runner, John Landy, the very next month, while running a race in Finland. Today, there are many runners who can run the four-minute mile, and it is no longer considered impossible.

So why was it considered impossible for someone to run a mile in less than four minutes? It was simply that it had not been done before. As soon as someone was able to do it, the mindset of others shifted, and their own limiting belief no longer stopped them.

You may have many limiting beliefs that are unnecessarily keeping you from your goals, but the good news is that these limitations are in your mind, and when you identify them, you can remove them. When dealing with limiting beliefs, you must reprogram your way of thinking in order to achieve what you want most in life.

I want to remind you, beautiful human, this has nothing to do with doing anything wrong, or what you should have been doing all along. Let's check the shoulda, coulda, wouldas at the door, and decide to move forward in a different way that serves you better. You did not know what you did not know, and now that you know, you can choose to take some action and make changes.

I had a client—let's call her Mary—who came to me because she decided it was time to make some major changes. The biggest change she wanted was a new job, because she was not satisfied with her current position. She felt stuck where she was because she did not have experience in other industries or in doing other roles. She knew that she was not fulfilled where she was but did not know where to begin. In addition to finding a new job, she wanted to spend time traveling the globe. (Does this sound like something that may have crossed your mind in the past? I know it has crossed my mind more than once.)

The first thing we had to do was identify her beliefs surrounding finding a new job she loved, in a role she wanted, and being able to travel. For her, they were not just beliefs; they were truths, and she had never looked at them in any other way.

The simple way to know if what you are thinking is a limiting belief is to ask yourself this question: "Is there anyone in the world who is doing what I desire to do?" An example would be, "I cannot go back to school because I have two children at home who depend on me." While having children can add extra considerations when it comes to doing something, you must ask the question: "Is there anyone in this world who has children and is going back to school to achieve an education?"

Another example is, "There are no eligible men or women in my city, and dating is impossible." Think of the message that is being sent into the world. Again, you can ask the question: "Are there women and men who are able to find their perfect mates in the city where you live?" Notice the change in how you feel when you ask such a question. To both of these questions, the answer is yes. Yes, there are parents who are going back to school; and yes, everyday city inhabitants are finding love in all different situations.

After identifying Mary's limiting beliefs surrounding finding her dream job in a totally new field, we also had to discover any other beliefs she would have that would keep her from her goal. Some of those included that she would not be able to leave her current job, she could not change careers, it would take too long, and that she could not choose an entirely new field. Once we removed all the beliefs that were blocking her, we set a goal for Mary that she would no longer be in her current job by May 1st, which was three months away, and that she would be able to travel for at least a month before starting her new position.

During the middle of March, Mary received notice from her boss that her position was being dissolved, and that her last day at the company would be April 30th. Suddenly forced to find a new job, a fire was lit under my client's derrière. She began connecting with people from her past and her present, and with people she had never met. She updated her résumé and sent it to anyone and everyone.

When you set a goal with intention, everything in the universe is going to come together to make sure that you achieve it. It does not always look the way you thought it would, so it is best to let go of how everything needs to come together. Soon after she received news about her position, I received a text message with Mary's itinerary for her trip to Sweden. It is the first vacation she had planned in years. This is an example of how the wheels get set in motion once we make a powerful declaration that we are going to do something, and begin taking the necessary action.

As a follow-up, when Mary returned from her trip around Europe, she began a new job, in a totally new field, that brings her more fulfillment than she thought was possible. It also provides her with more financial stability, which was one of her main goals in changing careers.

Since we are not in a coaching session in person, I am going to give you a simple exercise to help you identify the limiting beliefs blocking you, and help you loosen the grip they have on your unconscious mind so that it can begin focusing on making it happen rather than holding you back. Ready?

If you are ready to begin removing the obstacles that are keeping you from reaching your dream life, grab a pen and paper. Changing your life requires action, and only you can take the action to make it happen. This book is designed to be a do-with partnership. No amount of reading is going to bring your desired life closer to you, but if you take action now, you will reap the rewards later.

Okay, back to that piece of paper and a pen. At the top of the paper, write the area you want to focus on first. It does not need to be written in any particular format, and it can be only a few words. Some examples are a new job, a healthy romantic relationship, a trip to Thailand, earning $5,000 more each month, fitting into your favorite pair of jeans, a better relationship with your children, going back to school, getting into college, or any number of goals.

Once you have done that for one goal, create three columns on the page below the goal. In column one, write My limiting beliefs or decisions; in column two, write People in this world who are doing what I want to achieve; and in column three, write All the reasons I CAN attain this goal.

Example table:

My limiting beliefs or decisions	**People in this world who are doing what I want to achieve**	**All the reasons I CAN attain this goal**
I am not worthy of Success + my dreams/ happiness-	Carly Meyers Michelle Hillier. Countless other people.	I have the drive to do so. I have the tools + coaches there to help me.

After you have created the table, start with column one, filling out as many examples of limiting beliefs that are true for you. If you are struggling to find which limiting beliefs you have been holding onto, think about the last time you told someone what you wanted, and then followed up immediately with the excuse or excuses why you do not have it. Your excuses are thinly veiled, limiting beliefs.

It is important to not write down other people's beliefs. If there is something your mom, teachers, or friends used to say about the subject that do not ring true for you, do not add them. Focus on the beliefs that are stopping you, and that make you feel like achieving your dream may not be possible.

At this point, I need to remind you that your dream is not only possible, but it is your destiny. Your dream is the reason you were put on this Earth, and it is what is going to light you up and give you the energy to light up others in your life. Stay with the process, and keep taking steps towards achieving the life you were meant to live.

Once you fill out column one completely, move on to column two. It is important to note that if in a day, a week, or even a month, another limiting belief or decision pops into your head, add it to column one, and fill out the same process. For column two, take the time to look around you and see all the examples of other people of similar circumstance to you, who are taking action to do the things you want to do.

Recently, my husband suffered an injury that caused him to need major surgery. He is very athletic; playing rugby is a very large part of what brings him joy. He briefly let his mind wander to a place that was not serving him, and then decided to change his mind-set on what that surgery meant for his body, and for his future playing rugby. He began following Instagram accounts that showed other athletes coming back from the surgery, and how they were moving forward towards a healthy and strong body. He went online and read stories of people who have come back from injury. He made a specific plan of action on what was in his control to improve his outcome; and every day, he said a mantra to himself: "Every day, in every way, I am getting stronger, wiser, happier, and healthier."

This is just an example of how you can approach column two. It is important to choose people who are in a similar situation to you. If you choose Oprah or Beyoncé as an example in column two, you may end up with more limiting decisions. Look for people with similar lives; the only difference would be how they are taking action and making it happen. Once you have made a list of people who have done and are doing what you choose to do, it is time to move on to column three. Now, this is the most important column, so keep up your focus and dedication to this task, and bring it through to the end.

It can sometimes be easy to think of all the circumstances that are out of your control. It is often the first thing that comes to mind when a tough situation arises. There will be times that circumstances are out of your control, but you have a choice to either focus your attention on all the things you cannot control, or take the time to recalibrate your thinking to focus on ALL the many things that are in your control.

Think of your thoughts as noise going through a megaphone—the kind coaches use to talk to their team. When a coach wants to focus their attention towards a group of people, they face that group and point the megaphone towards them. If they want to focus their attention on another group, they turn their body and begin projecting in that direction. If they have their back turned toward the group they are trying to communicate with, nothing is reaching them, because they are not focusing their efforts towards the group they want to reach.

If your thoughts are focused on all the things that are out of your control, you are neglecting to put energy toward what will actually change the game for you and help you create your better future. The next time you catch yourself dwelling on what is not serving you, take a moment to thank yourself for the awareness of your thoughts; then reset your focus on what IS in your control. I would like to remind you—you beautiful, courageous, capable human—YOU have everything inside of you that you need to make it happen. Have fun with this list, and remind yourself of all the reasons why you absolutely can make your goal happen.

Inspired Thoughts

YOU CONTROL YOUR WAND OR IT WILL CONTROL YOU

"You can influence, direct and control your own environment. You can make your life what you want it to be."
- Napoleon Hill

So, who is in charge of your environment? Who is driving the life you are leading, and who is driving the changes you want to make? At my very first NLP training, one of the most profound lessons I ever learned was presented. It all begins with making the choice of to either be at cause or at effect in your life. What exactly does that mean? Let me break it down. A person who is at cause understands the role they play in their life. They know that their actions, emotions, and thoughts are the building blocks for what has shown up and what has not shown up in their life. When a problem arises, they take responsibility for it, and focus on how to change it. They understand that they have control of their destiny, and they can shape it the way they want with the right mindset and actions.

The other side of the coin is where most wishers, not achievers, live. When you become at effect of the environment around you, you give up control of your life, and you sit in the passenger seat. Often, I hear of various situations where someone or something else is causing a client to have the life they have. I hear that there is not enough time; they do not have the right resources; they have been wronged in the past. When you look at your life through this lens, you are taking yourself out of the game, and you become at effect of the circumstances around you. When you live this way, you are giving up control of your destiny.

When you are at cause for your life, taking responsibility for your actions, taking control of your time, efforts, attention, and thoughts, then you control the physical universe. When you are at effect of your surroundings and other people, then the physical universe is controlling you. Decide what kind of life you are going to lead; make the decision to take back control of your life, and create the circumstances that will bring you true fulfillment. Be more committed to your dreams than your struggle.

As my mentors like to say, "You can have reasons, or you can have results. Reasons are just excuses but results you can take to the bank."[3] The choice is yours. Remember, everyone starts from somewhere. It does not matter if you have been at cause your whole life or if you have let others drive your destiny for you. What does matter is how you choose to live your life moving forward from today. Have an honest conversation with yourself on which way you tend to live. Step by step, you will begin taking more control of your life, and you will begin to see how quickly you can achieve your goals when you make this one change. If you do nothing else but put yourself in the driver seat, you will see dramatic results. Think about it; how far can you drive a car from the passenger seat?

I will give you an example: I recently was in a session with someone I mentor. She is one of the smartest, most capable people I know, but sometimes she would get overwhelmed by the number of steps in her sales process that felt out of her control. There were elements that depended on other people, and it made her feel helpless in reaching the results that she desired. Because she felt like reaching her goal was not in her control, she was not able to see all the ways her mindset was contributing to being behind, and how shifting it would propel her towards achieving her goal. The simple act of white-boarding all of the parts of the process in her control helped her realize she had more control over the outcome than she thought.

Happiness Is a State of Being, Not a State of Having

◆ ◆ ◆

"Success is getting what you want.
Happiness is wanting what you get."
– Dale Carnegie

When you ask someone why they want what they want, they usually conclude that they are seeking happiness. Why do they want that new job? To make more money. Why do they want to make more money? To buy that new house they have been eye-balling. Why do they want to have that new house? To feel safe and secure. Why do they want to feel safe and secure? Because it will make them happy. If you follow most people's desires down a similar path, you will often reach a similar conclusion. Now, here is the catch: when you tie your happiness to material objects, you risk your happiness possibly being taken away.

If you focus your happiness on things that can never be taken away, you will find fulfillment—a glorious place to exist. Every day you wake up, the sun rises, you interact with people, you sip from cups, you speak on telephones, etc. These are all things that can easily be taken for granted if you do not pay attention to how truly wonderful each of those moments are. A few months ago, something happened that woke me up and caused me to realize how much I was taking for granted. It gave me the opportunity to reevaluate what made me happy.

One Sunday night, I thought the smoke I smelled was just my neighbors smoking a cigarette outside, and I thought nothing more of it. I went to bed as usual but was awakened at 4 A.M. with my room filled with smoke. It immediately became obvious that this was more than just my neighbors next door.

I opened my phone and looked to the news, where I saw

that there was a large wildfire burning forty-five minutes north of where I live. The fact that there was so much smoke in the air for a fire that was burning that far away put me on high alert immediately. I began to panic because my mom lives in the area where the wildfires were reported. I did everything I could to reach her by dialing her phone over and over, and sending multiple text messages. Finally, I reached her.

Her town was on fire, along with neighboring towns around her. It was the most shaken I had been in a long time. Luckily, my mom was able to evacuate safely to my house in San Francisco. Even though she left behind everything she owned, and every material item and keepsake she thought she cared about, she arrived in good spirits, with a grateful heart.

We sat down for a while, talking about what had been left behind and the items we could have gotten out of the house if given time. We both immediately realized that the once-cherished, material possessions truly meant very little when compared with her life and safety. And even though so much could not be replaced, these were just things at the end of the day.

After staying with me for a week, my mom was able to safely return to her home. Her home had been spared by this fire that took so much from so many people. I experienced a valuable reminder that week with her as we watched fires ravage the areas all around her home. My mom maintained good spirits and an attitude that she would be okay, no matter what happened. Now, that is not to say it would not have been incredibly hard, or incredibly sad, or other negative feelings, to have lost everything, but she had an air of peace, calm, and contentment throughout the week, while not knowing what her future would hold.

The reminder given to me was that it should not take almost losing everything for you to realize just how much you already have. If you were to take stock of the things that are most important to you in this life, how many of them would be material items? How many of them would have high price tags and designer labels? What is it that these material items are really bringing you? Is it security, power, or notoriety?

When you are able to focus your attention upon the non-material items in your life that you are grateful for, you will find a consistent sense of contentment that no one can take away from you. As a practical reminder, take the next five minutes or more to write down all the things in your life that bring a smile to your face, and that are not material possessions. If you are not able to get something quickly, close your eyes after reading this, and imagine the laughter of a child you care about. Hear his or her laugh with innocence and delight. Or imagine walking along the beach, with an ice cream in hand, on a hot day. What else brings you joy?

Things That Bring Me Joy

Kisses at the end of a text from a loved one. Walking along a beach front on a hot day - the waves kissing my feet. The feeling of the Sun on my back as I enjoy a chat + a cider w/ friends in a beer garden. Driving! Adventures. Having no time restrictions. Cooking a meal from Scratch then enjoying it. A chat over wine. A good waddle. A funny movie. First sip of fizz stick in the morning. A personal hand written note. A warm breeze of fresh air in nature. People laughing at my jokes.

The next time you feel a little lost, and you forget how much you have in this life, refer to this list, close your eyes, and focus your attention upon each one of these items. Even take the time to add more if you are in need of a reminder.

Magical Mission

◆ ◆ ◆

As we continue working through making changes to your life, I will assign tasks for you that will help you along your journey. It is entirely up to you to take action since, as we agreed when you began this book, action is required to make real changes. I hope you join me in another exercise today to take an additional positive step towards creating the life you want the most.

Today's task: Take five minutes to tell me about where you are with yourself right now. Pick an area of your life you would like to focus on first: relationship, career, personal growth, health, spirituality, etc. Spend five minutes telling me what is happening in this area of your life right now. Take a separate piece of paper and start writing now before reading ahead. No, really, no peeking!

Now that you have completed writing down your story, begin paying attention to how you tell your story. What words do you use? How do you describe your life? Who is writing your story? Now, look back at what you wrote down, and underline the areas where a circumstance, person, or situation was controlling your outcome, and circle all of the areas where you are taking total control. When it comes to what you have underlined, what can you do to take back control?

For example, let's say you are struggling with your weight, and you wrote, "I have issues maintaining my ideal weight because I do not have enough time to exercise or prepare healthy meals." In this example, you are blaming a lack of time for your health situation. Unfortunately, you will not be able to make the days longer than 24 hours, so what can you do to take control of that situation?

To take back control of your weight, you could start by

writing something like any of these examples: "I spend unnecessary time watching my favorite TV program; I can take that time, instead, to take a spin class. I can record my favorite show and watch it while jogging on a treadmill. I can walk to work instead of taking the bus. I can do squats between meetings."

When you begin taking control of your life, you make changes that create lasting benefits. When you take accountability for your actions, you also shift the energy to being at cause for your life, instead of at the effect of it, as we discussed earlier. It also changes the way you show up in this world. Once you have taken responsibility for your life, you begin to build your confidence and show up better for others in your life as well. Since how you do anything is how you do everything, when you learn how to do this in one area of your life, you begin to take control of other areas too. Let that sink in: How you do anything is how you do everything. That may be alarming as you consider how you currently do things, but you have the power to change anything and everything. The great news is when you begin showing up for yourself in one area of your life, the other areas begin to shift and transform towards what you want. The energy you put out towards your goals and others begins to change, and more of what you desire begins flowing into your life, because the walls you used to have up have begun crumbling down.

It does not matter if this has been your pattern for one day, ten years, or your entire life, because today, that pattern stops, and you get to take back control of your life. So be clear on what you want, and be ready to receive it in whatever form it shows up. We will get into more specifics on how to bring what you want into your life, in the chapters to come.

Inspired Thoughts

PRESTO CHANGO: COMMITTING TO YOUR DREAM

"The biggest adventure you can take is to live the life of your dreams."
- Oprah Winfrey

Where is it that you want to go? Where do you truly want to go? As mentioned in the previous section, it is important to know in which direction you are focusing your attention. Just like the GPS in your car, if your car is running and you point it in a specific destination, you will begin to move in that direction towards your end target. From time to time, you may go off course, but if your destination remains the end target, you will recalibrate your path and make your way back toward where you want to go. If you are sitting in the car, have not put anything into the GPS system, and have not bothered turning on the car, you cannot sit and wonder why you are not moving toward the destination you desire. In fact, you may just end up in that same location much longer than you wish. We both know you have places to go and people to see, so let's focus on how to make that happen.

There are two kinds of people in this world: those who believe in coincidences, and those who know that their thoughts, feelings, and actions steer the events in their lives. Have you ever had a thought about an old classmate, and then, out of the blue, he or she reaches out to you?

When this happens, do you exclaim, "What a coincidence! I was just thinking about you!" Or do you believe that you caused the meeting to happen by thinking about them? Or perhaps they were thinking about you, and that is what set into motion the accidental meet up. If you believe that your thoughts are energy sent out into the Universe, that they bring into motion what you are thinking about, then it is important to start paying attention to what is on your mind.

Goals Begin in the Mind

◆◆◆

"Whatever the mind can conceive and believe, the mind can achieve."
– Napoleon Hill

What you want to show up in real life first begins with what you create in your mind. Every invention ever created first began with a simple thought someone had, which grew into more complex thoughts, and then actions that were carried out. Law of Attraction experts, for years, have been letting you know that what you think about, you bring about. This also means that when you focus on what you do not want, you get more of what you do not want. That does not sound desirable, does it? When you focus upon what you appreciate and would like most, you create a different energy, and begin to receive what you want. Of course, it is a little more complicated than this, or every person who ever wanted a million dollars would be counting hundreds in the corner right now, and every person who thought something negative would be living a terrible existence. It is not as simple as thoughts becoming things, but everything you want does begin in the mind.

Here is a real-life example. If you wanted to have dinner with a friend somewhere healthy, you would not focus all your attention on what you did not want to eat. You would not look to your friend and say, "Well, I do not want a lot of grease; I do not want MSG; I do not want too much salt; and I do not want the food to be burnt." This does not help her understand what it is you do want to eat, so why does this happen so often when you speak about your dreams?

Instead, you should simply say, "I would love to eat somewhere healthy with lots of options." When it comes to things you know for a fact you can make happen, you have no problems stating your desires, and you do not allow what you do not want to even enter your awareness. This is because there is no resistance to the idea of getting a healthy meal if that is what you desire.

When it comes to items you are not sure you can attain, you tend to put more requirements on them, thus adding in more resistance. If you are not sure what I mean by resistance, take a moment to do this quick exercise. Without reading ahead, say out loud the following sentences, with five seconds in between each sentence:

1. I can easily create a situation that will bring 1 dollar into my life.
2. I can easily create a situation that will bring 10 dollars into my life.
3. I can easily create a situation that will bring 100 dollars into my life.
4. I can easily create a situation that will bring 1000 dollars into my life.
5. I can easily create a situation that will bring 10,000 dollars into my life.
6. I can easily create a situation that will bring 100,000 dollars into my life.
7. I can easily create a situation that will bring 1,000,000 dollars into my life.

Thank you for doing that exercise; you are getting pretty great at taking action. Now, as you read the first line, how did you feel? Pretty good, right? And you probably felt the same through the second and the third, and maybe even further. But for many of you, as you got further and further down the list, you may have begun to feel something different. A little voice inside your head that was beginning to talk back at you, telling you that it may or may not be possible, or maybe even a feeling in your body that felt heavy or different. That is resistance. It is the feeling of getting stuck, or that tightness that can hit your body. Read through it again and notice at which line you begin to feel a change in energy and body language. When it comes to learning how to focus your attention, it is important to not only keep your focus on what you want, but to also focus your thoughts on what feels free and good to you.

It is really important that you are not introducing more resistance to the process when you are creating goals, but it is also equally important that you do not cut yourself short and set BIG goals you want to reach. The rest of Part I is dedicated to how to create and execute goals that move you forward towards your dream life.

Magic exists in the physical plane, but it starts in the spiritual plane.

◆◆◆

Many years ago, I was in a relationship with a man who was less than perfect for me. I often felt neglected, confused, and unsure of where I stood in the relationship. It eventually ended, leaving me with a massive broken heart. I could not help but wonder whether it was me, and if all the nasty things he said at the end of the relationship had truth to them, or if he was just lashing out for other reasons. The truth is, it does not matter and, in the end, perception is projection anyhow. How I perceived the situation is truly only a reflection of what I was feeling about myself at that time. What does matter is how that experience created a shift in me and what I thought I needed in a relationship.

It was after this relationship that I began working with my coach to become clear on what I thought I wanted in a relationship. I realized that I had been living the same pattern over and over, and it was time I worked with a professional to help me understand what I was really looking for. I told my coach I wanted a man who was emotionally available, highly affectionate, and extremely in-touch with his emotions. Additionally, I wanted a man who was overly loving, so I never had to wonder what he was thinking, and I wanted him to be dedicated to me above all else.

I know how to manifest what I want, so I did. That man came exactly how I thought I wanted him. I immediately felt suffocated. I did not bring the man I needed my way; I brought the man I thought I wanted, because I was so influenced by my previous relationship.

How often do we create a picture in our mind of what we want, based on a previous experience that has driven us to crave the opposite? The point, my beautiful friend, is that it is not enough to be clear on what you think you want. First, you must let go of negative past experiences that may be influencing your vision of the life you choose, and then you can focus on discovering what you really want.

I am sure you are wondering how to let go of negative experiences. To begin, it is important to get to the bottom of

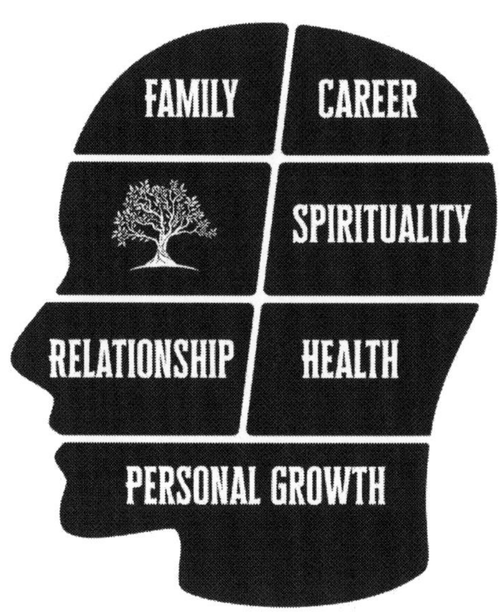

the motivation behind what you think you want. When you think about what is important to you about a given subject, I want you to ask yourself WHY that is important to you. Choose one area that you want to focus on first: relationship, career, personal development, family, health, or spirituality.

What is the most important aspect about that topic to you? Now, this can be tricky; it is not what you think SHOULD be important to you, or what others say is important about it, but what is important to YOU about that topic. The easiest way to know what is most important to you on any given topic is to ask yourself where you focus your time and attention. If you chose health as the topic, and you began making a list of what is important to you about health, and you had SLEEP at the top, yet you sleep only 5 hours a night, then SLEEP is not truly what is most important to you about health. If it is what you want to be most important to you, put a star next to it now, and we will revisit how to prioritize your life to get more of what you choose.

I did this exercise with my coach in regards to relationship. She asked me to write down everything that was most important to me about a relationship. I made an extensive list of 127 qualities I thought I needed in a man for my ideal relationship (please know you do not need to make a list this long; I just REALLY wanted to know where I was focusing my attention). After that, I cleared out all of what I did not want in a man, and removed my limiting beliefs (i.e. I was too old to find my perfect mate; no man could handle my success; I would not be able to travel as much if I were married, etc.).

Then, I looked deep into my heart and realized the one aspect I wanted in a man, above all others, was that he be interesting. My coach and I looked through my list of 127 qualities and saw that I had written this quality nowhere. It was such a shock! How could I have not known what was most important to me all along? As soon as I shifted my focus and attention on what I truly wanted in an ideal partner, he found me two days later. Could this have been a coincidence? Possibly, though I do not believe in coincidences. Regardless, now knowing what was really important to me, I was able to see him clearly, when in the past, I wouldn't have noticed the possibility.

By doing this exercise, you can begin to see if where you are placing your focus and energy will help you get to the outcome you desire. This is just one important step in the process. Before continuing to the next section, make sure you do the exercise.

- Write down what's most important to you about one specific area of your life (e.g., what's important to you about health? List ten things; they only need to be one-word answers or a short phrase).
- Then look at the list you made, and see if it: 1) matches the situation you are in now; 2) will get you the results you want. For example, if your number one value for career is working outdoors, and you are an investment banker, this might not lead to the greatest amount of fulfillment.
- Star the number one value for this area you are focusing on. When you make time later, elicit what's most important to you about the other areas of your life. This exercise will help you begin to identify what is most important to you, and if you are spending your time and energy in the areas that will give you the best results.

Making It Happen

◆◆◆

I believe that you can make a wish and have it come true

immediately. For many, this seems unlikely, because they expect it to also show up immediately. When you book a trip to Hawaii, you know for a fact that your trip will happen, and that in a short period of time, you will be sipping a Mai Tai on the beach. You do not doubt whether it will happen, because you have something in your hands, or at least your inbox, that you can see or touch. You rely on empirical evidence to let you believe it is possible, even if that trip is nine months out.

For wishes you make that do not have evidence you can see, smell, hear, or touch immediately, you start to create resistance, which causes it to move further and further away from you. Just as there is a physical process to booking a vacation, there is a mental process to follow that brings about your desired wishes. This process involves a few things to do before you begin taking action for a desired outcome. Often, you set out to achieve a desired goal, and it does not work out for one reason or another. This process is designed to make sure you are taking the steps necessary to achieve what you want, and that you are chasing the right types of goals to create fulfillment. Since you did the exercise earlier, you are clearer on what kinds of things are important to you. I am sure you have done plenty of exercises before, where you thought you were focusing on the right things to get the outcome you wanted, but it did not come to fruition because you may have been missing just a few key pieces. Spend some time thinking over each of the following key ideas; then, grab a pencil and paper, and begin taking notes on your personal goals.

The Keys to Inspired Outcomes[6]

◆ ◆ ◆

Key 1: State the goal in the positive. Does your internal dialogue tend to be positive or negative? You may be outwardly positive when speaking to others, but are negative, or even critical, when you speak to yourself. Think about how you have spoken to yourself over the last week; has it been mostly positive or mostly negative? Speak to yourself in the positive! For example, rather than stating your goal to not be unhealthy, instead say, "I want to be healthy," or better yet "I enjoy perfect health." There is another very important reason why this needs to be stated in the positive. Your unconscious mind, as brilliant as it is, cannot understand negatives. That is right, your UM simply cannot understand when you are using negatives in a sentence. If you say, I do not want to be late, your UM mind simply hears, I want to be late. So, for every area of life, say it how you want it. Now, take a moment and write down your goal, stated in the positive.

Key 2: Where are you now? Specify your present situation from your point of view. Try not to include what you have heard others say or express about your situation; this is all about you. If you do not know where you are, how can you begin moving towards where you want to be? Make sure, when you are writing this out, you are writing it from your point of view (i.e. I am currently....).

Key 3: Specify outcome. Spend some time thinking about what your desired outcome will entail. What will you see, hear, feel, think, etc., when you have it? Be thoughtful, and take some time to experience your desired outcome fully in your mind. Make it compelling. If it is something you truly want, there will be strong feelings associated with it. If, when you think about your desired outcome, no feelings are associated, ask yourself if this is truly what you want.

Key 4: Specify evidence. What will be the evidence that you have achieved your desired outcome? How will you know when you have it? What must happen for you to know that you have achieved your goal and reached the end? To go back to the example used earlier, how would you know you were taking a vacation? Is it when you decide on the location? Is it when you book the flight? For some, it is when you get to the airport, or maybe not until you get to the hotel at your destination. Really get clear on what the evidence will be, so that you know that you have reached the goal you want. Be specific.

Key 5: Be self-initiated and self-maintained. Why are you pursuing this? Are you doing it for someone else or for yourself? If you are doing something because someone else is telling you to do it, it will not work. This must be your desire, first and foremost. It also needs to be something that you are achieving yourself, and not relying on someone else.

Key 6: Will it produce the desired outcome? Many times, we set an intention for a goal, but do not think about what will actually happen when we get what we want. To make sure it is truly what you desire, go through the following questions, and be mindful of your response to each.

- For what purpose do you want this?
- What will you gain or lose if you have it?
- What will happen if you get it?
- What will not happen if you get it?
- What will happen if you do not get it?
- What will not happen if you do not get it?

If you have a strong desire to build a family, and yet your goal is to live in the mountains alone, these goals do not match up. Make sure to do this step to know if it will produce the desired outcome you want.

Key 7: Establish SMART goals. As you are about to embark on achieving your dream, set a few goals. In this case, make them SMART goals: Specific, Measurable, Achievable, Realistic, and Time bound. There are different ways people have looked at SMART goals. For our exercises, we will use the criteria above. A few reminders when you break this down: really take care to do this part with precision, starting with the specific portion. If you want to lose weight, instead of saying you want to lose 5lbs, say the end weight you'd like to be. If you want to make more money, instead of saying "more money," put a specific value on it. If you think about it, one penny more is "more money." What is the end amount you want to focus on? How will you measure your success? Is there a metric to follow? Is this a goal that is achievable, especially in the time-frame you set? When it comes to deciding if it is realistic, follow your internal compass, and do not sell your abilities short. Ignore the opinions of your friends and family if they have different opinions of what they think is possible, especially if the voices come from people who have never done what you are setting out to do. Finally, set a specific date when you are going to make this happen. Words matter. If you say in a month, a month will pass, and your goal will still be "in a month." Set a specific date, and hold yourself to it. You've got this!

Once you make a powerful declaration that you are going to do something, you set the wheels in motion to achieve your desires. Be clear on what you want, and be ready to receive it in whatever form it shows up. Often, when you get really clear about how you want to feel when you have achieved your goal, your unconscious mind finds what will bring that to you, and it may look a little different than you thought it would. That is OK! At the end of the day, it is all about finding what will bring you the most fulfillment and happiness. Take some time now to write down your goal in SMART format.

Key 8: Celebrate, celebrate, celebrate! Once you've achieved your goal, take the time to celebrate in a way that's meaningful to you. It doesn't matter if that's a simple dance around the living room, a spa retreat, a high five, or simply sitting in silence, feeling how amazing it is to reach your goal. Celebration keeps the inspiration flowing, and you taking action. As an added motivation, you can always write down how you'll celebrate once you get what you want.

In the last exercise, the first Key was to state your goal in the positive. Since your unconscious cannot process negatives, begin practicing stating what you want in the positive. Write down on note cards or on a piece of paper, "What do I want instead?" This will be a good reminder to mind your language and get into the habit of saying what you want, rather than what you do not want. A good one to start with is, "Remember." How often do you say, "Do not forget," and then that person forgets? Help yourself and others remember by stating it as, "Remember to…." And since you are probably a more advanced student, instead of saying the opposite of the negative thing you just said, really think about what you want instead. Instead of "I do not want to eat unhealthy foods tonight," say, "I cannot wait to eat foods that help my body thrive and make me feel great." You will soon get to the point where this is second nature.

Action, Action, Action

◆◆◆

Nothing in this world is created without taking appropriate action. Life rarely finds you or inspires you locked in your home waiting for something to happen. Remember my client, Mary, from earlier? She successfully achieved several life changes, including a new job in a new career, and multiple European vacations. Now that you have done the Keys to Inspired Outcomes exercise, I would like to take you through Mary's responses to the first five keys, so that you can identify strengths and opportunities in your own responses.

Key 1: Stated in the positive. When I asked Mary what she wanted, her initial response was, "I do not want to be stuck in this job." Her initial thought was negative! When you are focused on your problems, your thoughts are often negative. It takes mindfulness to create positive thoughts when dealing with an unpleasant situation. Not only was Mary's statement negative, but it was a very broad thought. When a desire is broadly stated, it is difficult to pursue a well-intentioned outcome. To take action on Mary's initial, negative thought, she could simply quit her job. Goal achieved? Well, she would no longer be stuck in the miserable job, but she would now be unemployed and without a plan of action. Instead, she refocused her thoughts to a positive statement and came up with this: "I want to work in the field of XYZ, with a job that will enable me to have work-life balance, and pays me at least X amount." As you know, she also added the positive thought that she would take a vacation to Europe. As you look back at your own step one, if it is not stated in the positive, please change it now. If you stated it in the positive the first time, excellent work! Taking this action now shows that you are ready to make some major changes.

Key 2: Where are you now? This one is your current situation as seen from your perspective. Mary stated that she was unhappy, overworked, and unmotivated with her current job. Her dissatisfaction was affecting relationships with family and friends.

Key 3: Specify outcome. Mary spent quite a bit of time working on this one. You will see that as you begin specifying the outcome you want, your ideas will flourish, so it is clever to set aside several hours, or even days, to let the thoughts come. Mary visualized herself walking into her new job (whatever it would be), in a relaxed, content manner. She saw that her shoulders were visibly relaxed, and she felt a calm, yet excited energy. She heard herself speaking enthusiastically about the workweek ahead, and even singing as she got ready in the mornings. She saw the teamwork during meetings, and could hear the sound of collaboration, something that gave her a really good feeling. She envisioned cheerful family meals, where everyone shared and laughed together.

Additionally, she stated the income she would make at her new job. She also knew that this new job would allow her to pursue innovative ideas within this field, and that she would have work-life balance. For Mary, this meant that she would work 40 hours per week and be able to take at least two long vacations a year.

She also saw, felt, and heard that European vacation. When doing this process, she really felt herself being in that really good place, and felt the feelings she would feel when she had all of it. This was how she really knew this was what she truly desired.

Key 4: Specify evidence. Now, this is a very important step that needs to be specific. For Mary, she knew that she had accomplished her goal of getting her dream job when she was sitting at her desk in her home office, holding a copy of her offer letter, which included all the specific requirements she desired. Once she had that offer letter in her hand, she knew her goal had been met. For some people, in a similar situation, it may be the verbal confirmation that they got the job from a recruiter. For others, it could be walking in the door of the new office on their first day. For some, it could be seeing that first paycheck in their hands, or maybe telling their family they got that new job. For the goal you are looking to reach, what is the specific evidence that you need to KNOW for certain that you have achieved your goal? Once you have that evidence written down, and you take the time to really visualize yourself with that evidence, if you do not feel the way you want to feel when you have it, find better evidence for you.

Key 5: Be self-initiated. There are people in your life who want what is best for you and will give you their recommendations and suggestions. This is fine, but if the goal you are working on is not one that you chose because it is not what YOU truly want, then this is not the process to obtain it. How often do you see others doing something to please another, or trying to do something because it is what their spouse, partner, or family member wanted? There is not the same level of passion and desire behind it, and as we mentioned earlier, the conscious mind is the goal setter and the unconscious mind is the goal getter. If your unconscious mind did not instigate this change, then you do not have the pieces in place to make sure you get what you want. As you look at your goal, make sure that it is truly what you desire, and it is something that you, yourself, can work to make happen.

Key 6: Will it produce the desired outcome? Yes! Taking this action and making this change would allow Mary more freedom to spend time how she wanted, and challenge her to learn a totally new role in an exciting industry.

Key 7: When I first learned about SMART goals, I was told to always put my name in the goal so there would be no doubt who I wanted this goal for. For Mary, it looked like this:

"It is now May 1, 2017, and I, Mary Magic, have now accepted an offer to work in X role, with a salary of more than $100,000 a year, with full benefits and at least three weeks off paid leave each year. I work with a collaborative team, and I enjoy coming into work, and feel fulfilled."

It's important to note that she didn't specify what company she had to work for. This allowed for more possibility, and sometimes the best fit comes from a place we didn't even know existed. All that really mattered to her was that her primary desires were met so she would have a career that she felt fulfilled in.

Key 8: Celebrate! What better way to celebrate than a

trip to Sweden?

As you have undoubtedly determined, Mary put an abundance of time and energy into working through the Keys to Inspired Outcomes. She may have begun with a few rash thoughts, but she worked through them until they evolved into astute, attainable goals. I encourage you to do the same. Take what you have started with, and allow your thoughts to percolate and evolve.

It is your turn to create change in your life. In this moment, decide where you are in your life. Are you at a seven out of ten? Four? Nine? Wherever you are, ask yourself what the one thing is that you can change, to move up to the next level. Is it your health, your relationship, a new career, or something else? Once you do that, see if it meets the keys to an inspired outcome. If it does, great! Move forward! If it does not, choose another desired outcome. Creating life change is a process that you can begin immediately. If only you could close your eyes, make a wish, then open them to see it unfold before you. Magical things occur during the process, so do not delay; act now. I will be with you through this entire process, as your guide. Believe in yourself, and keep learning and evolving as you follow this path.

Dreams do come true

◆◆◆

I am a daydreamer. I love taking moments of silence and thinking about all of the distant places I want to visit, and all of the experiences I want in my life. My mother is from

Asia, and while I have always wanted to go, I believed for a long time that it was too expensive of a trip to make anytime soon. After working with my coach to remove the limiting beliefs that were blocking me in my life, I realized that anything is possible, and sometimes a great outcome will come from a direction totally different than I thought. A few years ago, while at a conference, I saw there was a business class trip to Asia, for two, being given away for a $10 raffle. A luxury hotel was also included! I felt in my bones that trip was meant for me, so I bought a ticket. My colleagues, who

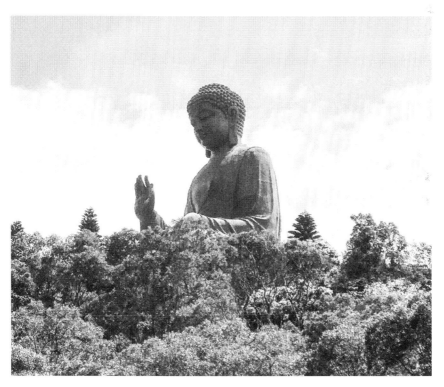

This is a photo I took, on Lantau Island, of the largest bronze Buddha statue in the world.

were also in attendance, gave me many reasons why I was not going to win. They pointed out that there were 8,000 people attending the conference, and that the odds were not in my favor. They told me that they never win anything at all. The reasons kept coming and coming, but my heart did not change. I felt that I would win. I somehow knew that I would win. So, I bought the ticket, and I won a trip to Hong Kong. When they called my name over the loudspeaker, my heart leapt, and I was beyond excited.

All things are possible when you believe that they are possible. I was not jaded to believe I would never win. Instead, I put myself in the game because, in my heart, I was connected to the outcome. I also allowed myself to envision

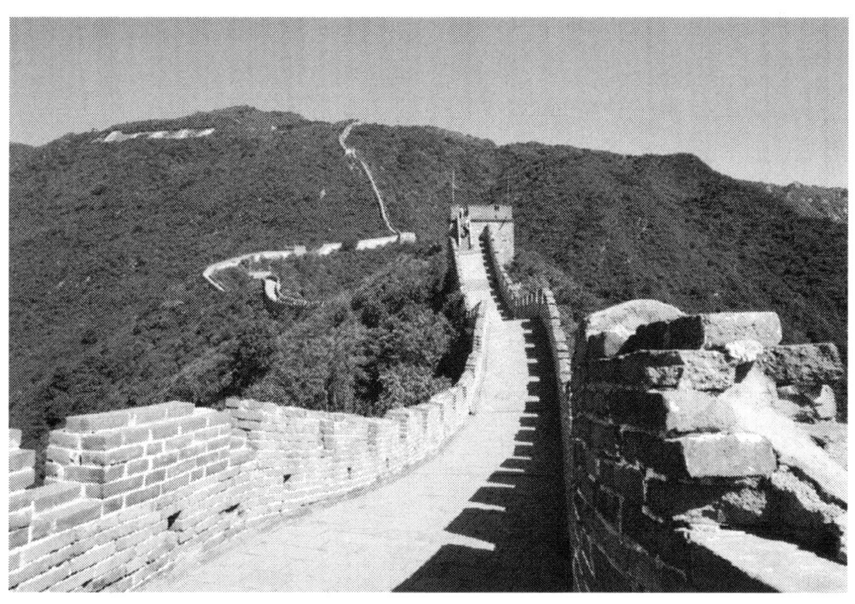

Photo taken from Trip #2 to Beijing and the Great Wall of China

myself on that trip; I saw them calling out my name, and I began thinking about when the ideal time would be to go. I had such faith that this could be mine that I pulled up the directory of everyone in attendance and made sure I was the only Michelle Hillier in attendance, so that when my name was called, I would be sure it was me they were speaking about. I tapped into the magic of what I wanted to create. I wanted that trip to Asia!

The next year, at that same conference, the same raffle fundraiser was happening. After seeing my results the year before, I thought all of my colleagues would jump at the chance to support the charity and possibly win an incredible trip.

Maybe they have not won in the past, so they thought it was not possible now. Maybe they were simply adopting the thoughts and opinions of those around them. Or, possibly, they never conceived of getting to Asia because of a raffle, and they only focused on buying an expensive plane ticket and booking an expensive hotel. Whatever the case may be, when people focus on thinking only about what they want and not seeing results, it is directly matched with the fact that there is probably just as much, or even more, going against whatever he or she is putting out into the world.

If the current going against the goal is stronger than the current flowing towards the goal, life will not change, and could even go against it. The trouble is that people often believe they are doing everything possible to get what they want, and oftentimes they truly believe their thoughts are aligned with their desires.

At first, the flow is easy. A challenge arises that creates a desire for something different. A major disagreement with a manager can spark the desire to find a different job opportunity. There is no real resistance there, because the idea of getting a new job—any job—can feel plausible and easy.

The next thought may be, in what industry do I want to work? What company do I want to work for? What role do I want? As the monkey mind begins (that fast-paced chatter that begins on a loop inside your mind without real focus), and you spiral deep down into specifics, more and more resistance may begin popping up. Resistance could be in the form of negative emotions, negative thoughts, limiting beliefs, doubts, etc. The details are where your mind can start to push back on the desire you want to focus on.

This is true in every area of life, including when you are having disagreements with others. Imagine you are with your significant other, and you both are really hungry (having a conversation while hangry is never a good idea), and you decide you want to go out to dinner. At this point, you are in total agreement with one another. You choose your favorite Greek spot, and he chooses his favorite Mexican, and this is where the contrast begins. When you got into the details, the disagreement began, but if you take it a little higher and a little vaguer on why you each chose what you chose, it turns out he is craving spicy food, and you really want a salad. With this information, you decide on Thai: he can get all the spicy food he wants, and you love their papaya salad.

It is hard to get in disagreement when you are high-level on a topic. Try this next time you are having a conversation with someone you disagree with, and see if in the end you both actually want the same outcome. Then you can find a different way to work together.

When it comes to getting what you dream about, loosening the grasp on the outcome opens the range of magic around you. For another example, let us suppose you want to buy a new car. You get really excited at the prospect, and it feels light and fun. Then you decide on the make, then the model, and maybe you even begin to choose the color and all of the other details you decide you must have in a car.

Now, the ways in which you can get that car become limited, because you need to seek out the specific dealership that carries the very specific make, model, color, and accessories you want. The fun can begin to fade as you limit your options, and then the dreaded "hows" begin creeping in. How am I going to find this exact car; how will I pay for the car I want; how will I find it in time, etc.

Removing the limitation of certain specifics opens a greater area and space to create magic. This is the difference between focusing with your head (the car must be blue) and focusing with your heart (driving it must feel good). And when you open up to other possibilities, more options come your way, which you did not even think of in the first place. Allow for even better things to come into your life, and from a direction you never would have guessed.

As you practice, you will begin to get very good at feeling

your way through your goals, and allowing them to show up in wonderful and new ways. The key is, when it arrives, to have gratitude for it. Energetically rejecting an outcome that is not exactly how you wanted is not a great way to show the world you appreciate what it provides.

Celebrate those moments instead, and see more and more of what you desire come your way. If something shows up completely different from what you wanted, take a moment to see what energy and intentions you put out into the world, and what actions you did not take that could have changed the outcome. Then, adjust and learn for the future. It is all about learning how to pivot and be flexible, as you grow into a smarter, stronger, and more incredible you.

Inspired Thoughts

CASTING MAGIC SPELLS: WHY WORDS REALLY MATTER

In this first part, we have discussed the role that your mindset plays in achieving your goals and putting into motion the life you want to live. Real magic truly is done with the power of the mind. People cast spells every day and never realize they are doing it. The words you speak, and even the words you think, are powerful, and can set things in motion. As children, we heard the old rhyme, "Sticks and stones …." You know how it goes, though words can hurt you, and they can heal you. Words are powerful! Words carry incredible weight and meaning; they can either do what you intend or, if you change them slightly, the outcome will change. The thoughts in your head become the words that you speak; the words you speak change how you feel and, ultimately, become the actions you take. Think about the last time you thought you may be getting sick. Once you said it out loud, did you notice symptoms that really were not there before? From that point, you started to feel worse, even though, shortly before, you did not feel so bad. This is even worse when someone else suggests you may be getting ill, and you take on that thought! That negative suggestion you made to your body began to set in motion how you were treating your body and how it responded. By changing that one phrase to, "My body is temporarily getting an immune system boost," may cause you to treat your body differently, and add some healthier practices into the mix. Whatever it is you want, really put into practice using the words in your mind and in your life that will bring that about.

There is no ambiguity when it comes to how you are feeling, and that is the magic trick for knowing what you are genuinely gravitating towards. If something in your life makes you consistently smile when recalled, those are positive thoughts. When you find yourself grimacing at a thought or idea, there are negative thoughts underneath it all. You may believe you are thinking of something positive that will benefit you, but if you find yourself grimacing, sighing, or furrowing your eyebrows when you think about it, think again. Do not try to fool your unconscious mind; your results will be based on your real thoughts and feelings. Think of all of the times you were leading with your head and not getting the results you wanted, and in your heart, you knew it was for the best. Follow your heart. The right path is not always about finding the easiest way; it is about finding what you are made of, and learning how to triumph over doubts and missteps. Sometimes a leap of faith feels major, but little do you know that there is a clear bridge under you, waiting to help you along to the other side, should you ever need it. And fortunately for you, you have the strength to fly while dancing on water, so you do not have to choose between the clouds and the ocean. This is only the beginning for you; there are so many more beautiful adventures ahead for you. Stay on the path, and you will create the change you want in your life.

Before you move onto the next section, I encourage you to do the exercises in Part One. Really take the time to get clear about what it is you want from this life and what you want to give to this world. Every flame begins with just a little spark, and should you choose it, you can bring all the power you desire to your life.

Inspired Thoughts

PART TWO - BODY

"The first wealth is health."
– Ralph Waldo Emerson

In part one, we went through the ways you can focus your mind to achieve desired results. Everything we create first begins in the mind, and then it is put into action. As you continue to create healthy self-talk, and focus your thoughts on what you want most out of life, you will begin to see your dream life show up in ways you did not know were possible. Changing behaviors and processes takes time and dedication. I know you have it in you to begin living a healthier, happier, and more fulfilled life. When you show up as your happiest and healthiest self, you show up a more complete person for others in your life.

Now that you have taken strides to improve your mindset, it is time to dive into how to create a healthy lifestyle that will allow you to grow your physical magic and share it with others.

Even though this book is divided into sections, separating the mind and body, they are very much connected. The mind-body connection has been discussed in countless books and studies, though how often do we really take the time to connect with our bodies, check-in, and fully assess our state of health? How often do we take for granted the fact that we ask this beautiful body of ours to do so many things for us throughout the day, and rarely thank it. We definitely give it criticism when it does not perform 100% the way we want it to. What would happen if we slowed down and practiced more self-care and gratitude for our beautiful bodies? Even when they are at their worst, they are still doing what they can to get you through the day. And ultimately, what shape our bodies are in are a direct correlation with our thoughts, what we put into it, and other factors we contributed.

There are so many reasons why creating the healthiest version of yourself is in your best interest. For example, when you are well rested, you have the energy to bring your A-game to taking care of your family, crushing your career goals, and/or enjoying surfing on that Tahitian vacation. When you are calm, you are able to see so many possibilities not available to you when you are highly stressed. If you are already on top of your health game, bravo! You will still be able to learn a few tips and tricks in this section, so keep following along, take what calls to you, and leave behind anything that you have already mastered. If you have ignored your health for a while, and made the oh-so common claim, "I'll exercise more when I have time," or, "I'll eat healthy when I can afford organic foods," or, "I'll start meditating when life calms down..." If you are so busy that you cannot focus on your health, this is precisely the time to take back control of your body. There are endless ways to begin taking care of your body. Why not start at the very beginning?

Inspired Thoughts

EXTRAORDINARY ENERGY: SLEEPING BEAUTY AND ENCHANTING MORNINGS

"Efficiency is doing things right, effectiveness is doing the right things."
– Peter Drucker

How you do anything is how you do everything. If you are always on time for meetings, you are most likely always on time to meet with friends and family. If you are clean and organized at work, then you are most likely clean and organized at home as well. If you are lazy in love, you may be lazy in other areas. And if you wake up and rush chaotically through your mornings, then there is a good chance that the rest of your day follows a similar pattern. Every day, when you wake up, there is a new opportunity to improve the way you spend your day. Imagine waking up refreshed, alert, and ready to take on the day. How would that change the way you enter your first interactions with loved ones, your morning meetings, or whatever task you take on first?

Everyone wishes to wake up feeling refreshed and energized for the coming day, but refreshed mornings begin with your nighttime routine. Did you get a good night's sleep last night? Do you sleep well most nights? If you usually wake up feeling groggy and tired, then you may not be able to get the most out of your day. We all hear that we need eight hours of sleep each night, but have you ever thought about why?

During sleep, your body regenerates, rebuilds, and repairs cells. The pineal gland, located in the brain, receives information through light. As the sun sets, or lights are dimmed, this gland senses the change and begins to secrete a hormone, melatonin, to prepare your body for sleep. Think of the pineal gland as your internal clock. Even though we all have this internal clock, most of you focus on the time on your watch or your phone, rather than what your body is trying to tell you.

Typically, melatonin levels begin to rise a couple of hours after sunset, and let your body know that it is time to sleep. Do you go to bed two hours after sunset? Or are you still awake at midnight? Unfortunately, the bright light from technology prevents the secretion of melatonin, and most of us spend our evenings watching television or tablet screens, or we're reading, working, or just hanging out under overhead lights. If you have occasional insomnia, or wake up feeling groggy much of the time, consider a different bedtime routine. To put it simply, that late night social media and last-minute emails are messing up your sleep rhythms, and creating a harder environment for peaceful sleep.

Skip the screen at least an hour before you go to sleep; opt for a book, meditation, or old fashioned conversations. Whenever you are starting a new routine, it is important to be patient with yourself. If you have been watching TV until you fall asleep, for the past decade, stopping cold turkey is an option, but it is not the only option. Choose one day the first week, where you read a book for fun or write in a journal. Build upon that routine until you have created a totally new way of going to bed. It is not about being perfect or doing something 100% right the first time; it is about doing the best you can, day by day, until it becomes second nature. It does not matter how slow you go, so long as you do not stop. A week from now, a month from now, even a year from now, think about where you will be in your life if you start today.

Quieting the Monkey Mind

◆ ◆ ◆

Another reason why you find it hard to sleep is that you may have chatter in your head, keeping you from falling asleep or falling back to sleep if you wake up in the middle of the night. Anytime you have unresolved thoughts or actions, your body and mind are being drained of energy while focusing on what is unresolved. Oftentimes, this unresolved thinking is caused by thinking of everything you need to do the next day.

In order to allow your mind to let go of that thought

pattern for the night, take a sheet of paper and write down the top three to five most important things you need to accomplish the next day, and when you will accomplish each task. Giving your mind structure and focus will help you let go of thinking about it for the night.

If you still have unresolved chatter in your mind, take this exercise a step further by visualizing how you will feel 15 minutes past the successful completion of each of those tasks. Remember, your unconscious mind cannot distinguish between what is real and what is pretend. If you put yourself in the feeling of successfully completing that task, your mind will mark it as resolved, and you will be able to get some rest. Once you have rested, you are in a better position to take on each of those tasks, and you may even see opportunities on how to complete them based on what you visualized the night before.

Mindful Mornings

◆ ◆ ◆

When it is time to wake up, do you experience morning madness? Do you hit the snooze button, and then drag yourself out of bed to begin a mad dash to get to work on time? Like a race, how you start will determine your level of success. You do not want to wake up already behind, and spend your morning playing a game of constant catch-up. If you do, you could always be chasing after success but never quite reaching it.

What would your ideal morning feel and look like? What

would be the pace and energy of a morning well spent, and what all could you accomplish? Decide that you are going to take back your mornings, and wake up on your terms, feeling refreshed and ready to face the day. You want to set a pace for your day that allows you to enjoy yourself and feel good throughout the entire day. Take a few moments at the beginning of each day, before you get out of bed, to assess and listen to your body. Give yourself a little bit of time to begin feeling present and aware of your body and surroundings. Start wiggling your fingers and wiggling your toes, while taking in big, deep breaths to bring new energy to your body. Now that you have a little time to wake up and spend time checking in with yourself, it is time to get out of bed.

Do you head straight for the coffee pot? Do not worry; if you are an avid coffee consumer, I will not attempt to eradicate it from your life. However, I will implore you to drink a glass of warm water before you have the coffee. At night, your breathing depletes you of hydration, so when you wake, restoring your hydration level will help wake you and give you a morning boost. Oftentimes, that grogginess you feel is in fact dehydration, and by rehydrating the body, you may not even need that morning cup of Joe. Additionally, drinking water has been shown to aid in flushing out toxins, jump starting your digestive system and increasing your metabolism.

While you are sipping your warm water, what are you thinking? To be more specific, what are the first words you say to yourself when you wake up? While you sleep, you are able to pause any attention and thought on the issues that may be troubling you. When you wake, it is an opportunity to set the tone for the day, and to set an intention for how you want the day to go.

Morning Energy Exercise

◆◆◆

Over the years, I have taken many courses and masterminds, had many coaches, and tried many different morning routines and techniques. The following exercise is one that always resonated with me, and takes only a few minutes. If you are looking to try a new morning exercise, give this one a try, or create your own take on the activity below.

When you first wake up, the part of your brain that can talk you out of what is possible is still a little bit sleepy. Take this as an opportunity to create the energy you desire most, and send it out into the world to connect with the people, places, and things that can bring your dreams to you.

Start by lying on your back and connecting with your breath. You have just woken up, so take a few moments to deeply breathe in and exhale out, while you begin to wiggle your fingers and toes to gently wake the body. Next, you want to visualize a ball of energy floating right above your chest. My ball is golden and shines brightly, but you choose the color that gives you the most feeling. If your ball is a muted blue, and that stirs happy feelings within you, then please use that color. If bright neon green brings you joy, then use that. Once you have your ball of energy, place your hands on each side of the visualized ball. I imagine mine is the size of a basketball, so I have my hands roughly one foot apart. Now is the time to use that beautiful imagination you have.

Begin to visualize the area of your life you want to focus the most attention on. If it is relationship, I want you to feel the way you would feel when you have the relationship you desire most. It is not about creating the specifics of what it will look and sound like, but getting into the feeling of how you will feel when you have what you desire. If you need to visualize or imagine hearing something specific to get you to that feeling, go for it! Once you have a strong feeling the way you want, then imagine that ball of energy growing and filling the room. Then, visualize it filling your home, and imagine it growing and filling the block. Now let it grow until it is as big as the city, the country, and the world, and then, finally, imagine sending that energy out into the entire universe. Allow yourself a minute to ask that energy to connect you to the people, places, and things that will allow you to step into the situation that will bring you that feeling you just sent out.

Because your physiology can play into how you feel, do this exercise with a big smile on your face, if it helps you get more emotion out of the exercise. Set an intention to try this exercise once this week. Notice how it helps shape your morning and how you feel as you wake. For those of you who do not make time for yourself in the morning, set your alarm five minutes earlier, and make a choice to do something different to help you achieve a different result.

Use Your Body Language to Give You Power

◆ ◆ ◆

We have all heard that our body language communicates with others, but have you ever thought about how your body language communicates with you? Now that we have begun a morning routine that will help set you up for a more successful day, let's take it a step further than your imagination and mindset. Have you ever noticed your body language as you get out of bed in the morning? Do you spring into action, or do you drag yourself out of bed and slump around the house? I realize that not everyone is a morning person. In fact, I was never a morning person. I used to have many alarms set to try and get myself going in the morning. I even had one across the room that I would get up, hit snooze on, and then crawl back into bed. Part of it was that I was not excited to go to wherever I was going, and we will work on that in the next section. Part of it was that I was still in a haze, thinking of everything I had to do that day; but mostly, it was all I had ever known. My body language in the morning was mimicking someone who is timidly entering into the day, without much confidence or purpose. I am not suggesting that you need to jump into action first thing in the morning, but there is a simple exercise that can help boost your energy and mentally set you on the right path for a wonderful day.

Channel Your Inner Superhero

◆◆◆

You have gotten out of bed after your energy exercise, and it is time to take your first steps into the day. If you choose to make the time, take two minutes to greet the day like a superhero. Stretch your arms high overhead and take in a deep breath. Expel all the sleepiness out of your body, and plant your feet firmly on the ground. Connect with the ground; draw stability from it. Now, firmly place your hands on your hips, raise your head high, and elongate your body so that your chest rises and your shoulders are drawn back and down, away from your ears. Now, put a giant smile on your face. Even if you do not think you have anything to smile about, put one on your face anyhow. When you put yourself into this pose, and hold it for at least one minute, you will begin to release messages to your brain, of confidence, poise, and joy. You are the superhero of your day, and you get to create the outcomes you desire.

You can use this posture and process at any point during the day. Have a big meeting? Go into a room, or the bathroom, and stand in this pose with a smile on your face, for one minute before you enter your meeting. Have a first date you are nervous about? Give this a go. In fact, you can use this trick anytime you need a confidence boost, or to ground yourself. Set a goal to do this at least one morning this week, and see how you feel. Since you are in the take-action mindset while reading this book, take a minute now to put the book down and do this exercise. If you are in the room with other people, go ahead and have them do it with you. Life is meant to be fun, so play!

Now you have some new tools and tricks to help you get your day going in the right way. Play with these processes and see which ones work best for you. As mentioned in previous sections, all habits are created through repetition and practice. If mornings have not been your most lively time of day, it is okay to start with just one of the suggestions above.

Start slow and build up to a routine that maximizes your day. But no matter whether you are traditionally a morning person or not, you picked up this book to change your life, so make the choice to try something new, and dedicate yourself to the behaviors that will help change the course of your life for the better. I know you can!

Inspired Thoughts

When It Doesn't Work Like a Charm: Getting Rid of What No Longer Serves You

A young woman, who has always wanted to become a cyclist, decides today is the day! She heads out and buys a road bike, and every piece of biking gear the shop sells. She puts on her new jersey, padded bike shorts, and the clip-in shoes, then ties her hair back, grabs her helmet and water bottle, then grabs another water bottle, and then another, as she thinks she will be incredibly thirsty. Then she grabs the new cycling backpack and starts filling it with other necessities, just in case. She throws in a sweater and a pair of jeans, in case she wants to eat brunch after her ride. What if her phone runs out of battery? She decides that she must bring her extra-large back-up charger. She climbs clumsily onto the bike, trying to balance all the items she believes she needs with her, and after about four blocks, she gives up, turns back, and has no idea why she was not able to ride like the wind.

The exuberant would-be cyclist overwhelmed herself with unnecessary clutter, and ended up holding herself back. If you were running a marathon, would you bring extra socks, just in case? Would you see how many hair bands you could get in your hair, or layer on extra pieces of clothing? No, you would wear what you need, and not one thing more.

Clearing out the Clutter and Creating Clarity out of Chaos

◆◆◆

The key to quick action is to keep it simple and manageable. Down the line, you can begin to bring more into your process if you choose, but it is unnecessary. Keep it simple, and you will go far. If you have a meticulously kept space, amazing! When you clear out your space, you create room to design your ideal life, and give yourself more mental clarity and energy.

Is your home or workspace set up like our cyclist's backpack? Do you have everything you may ever need to access, sitting on top of your desk or your kitchen counter? If you have organized chaos, or chaos-chaos, maybe it is time for a little space reset. When you have a ton of clutter in your home, you stop energy from free-flowing around you. A cluttered environment also clutters the mind, causing undue stress and anxiety. Remember earlier about how the brain is drained of energy when it is dealing with unresolved situations? An unorganized area can drain the brain unnecessarily, and take precious focus away from the magic you could be creating.

Clearing your space and making an accessible area to learn, work, and create will increase your productivity and lower your stress levels. It also makes it very easy to take note of all you already have, and brings a sense of fulfillment, minimizing the desire to purchase more. Ready to make some room for more of what you want to show up in your life?

Ask yourself the following questions, and then we will embark on a little exercise in clutter clearing: What is the first thing you see when you open your eyes? Can you walk easily through your rooms? Is there blocked energy throughout the house? Do the colors you see bring you joy? What is your initial reaction to your surroundings as you open your eyes?

As you went through those questions, what items caught your attention? It is time to focus on those items that create clutter and keep you from having more of what you want. For each one, ask the following questions to determine whether the item should stay or go.

- Does this item give me joy?
- Does this item feel good on my body?
- When was the last time I used this?
- Does this have sentimental value?

- If I never saw this again, would I even notice?
- Does this item bring up sad or hurt feelings or thoughts?
- Do I have something similar to this already?

If the item in question does not meet your requirements to keep it, set it in a box to donate, sell, toss, recycle, or gift to someone. Start this process in the area of the house that you feel needs the most help first. To begin clearing energy more quickly, start with the physically largest items in the room, and you will immediately begin clearing space.

When you looked at the things that you own, and noticed that you have duplicates of many of them, did you realize that you are energetically sending out into the universe the idea that you think nothing more can come your way? Holding on to everything you have (even multiple versions) indicates that you believe receiving more may not be possible. Your clutter communicates a great deal about what you believe.

How do the things around you make you feel? Sometimes we become accustomed to our belongings and do not realize the impact they have on us. A fitting example of this emotional impact is photos you have in your space. Some old photos may harbor unpleasant memories if they cause you to recall a person, a time, or a place. You may also have gifts or other items from a past relationship that have become a part of your space. Photos and other objects connect energy from past relationships to you. You may no longer be the person you were when you received those items, and keeping them around tethers you to a person you no longer are. If you cannot part with something that is very sentimental, even though it can bring up negative memories, place it in a box out of sight.

You can also make an unwelcome environment for guests when they come over, or worse, create a circumstance where you do not feel comfortable having guests into your space, your home, and your life. When you shut people out, you are shutting out opportunity.

Another area where clutter causes issues is in the workplace. Are you keeping your space orderly? If your workspace is cluttered, it likely slows down your productivity, as you must constantly stop to search for things or move things around to make room. And since perception is reality, it can also create a perception of you with colleagues and customers, which may not be accurate.

What do you do with the things you have? Do you rent extra space to store the items you are holding on to? The cost of storing things can add up over time and become a financial burden; whereas selling or donating these things may bring financial gain. I hope you will consider the impact your surroundings have upon you and your guests. When you clear out the clutter, clarity emerges.

You will be amazed at how ideas and energy begin to flow! Your energy levels will be higher, and your stress levels will be lower. Is that not the goal, after all? If there are items that you cannot seem to let go of, which you know serve no purpose, ask yourself why. Is that concert ticket, from the first date with that person from that troubled relationship, really something you need to keep in your life? Sure, many times these items represent the best of the times we had with certain people, but that does not mean keeping it will bring those feelings back, and oftentimes it does the opposite.

Holding onto items that do not serve any purpose or bring you joy can energetically show a lack mentality. When you begin to discover why you are holding onto possessions that could be blocking your growth, write them down. These could be limiting beliefs that are stopping you, and you can use the process in part one to get rid of them and move on towards what you want instead.

Disconnect from Technology

◆◆◆

A few years ago, I took a trip to Rome. I took an overnight flight and landed in Italy at 7 AM; I had not slept one bit. Arriving at the hotel, all I could think of was a large cappuccino, and maybe some food to eat, before crashing in my room for a nice, long nap. What I got was so much more than I could have imagined.

I arrived at the hotel several hours before I was able to check-in, so there went my thoughts of a nap. An incredibly kind man (who happened to look like a Roman god) at the front desk led me upstairs to a balcony, where the Pope used to take his morning tea. I sat there feeling the cool breeze, listening to the bells in the distance, and ordered a cappuccino. I sat, taking deep breaths, feeling the cool morning Italian air course around me, and felt at peace. Even the touch of the white linen that covered my table felt extra special as I allowed my hands to take in everything around me. I consider myself fortunate to have been reminded how lucky I was to be on this earth experiencing a new city.

Suddenly, a group of very exuberant Italians burst through the door. This group consisted of all ages, the youngest being around four years old, and the oldest being possibly in his 80s. They were all smiles and laughed together as they came into the area where I was sitting; they were enthusiastic about spending time with one another. I could not help but notice that there was not one cell phone in sight. No one had a computer, e-reader, tablet, or any kind of technology to distract them from spending time with one another during this precious breakfast. They were there to spend time in each other's company, and that is where all of their attention was focused.

For two hours, I was in the presence of their laughter and their lively storytelling as they ate in genuine glee. At no point did someone pull out their cell phone to update their status or take a selfie. No one was checking to see what else was happening in the world. They were present, 100%, with each other. It was so refreshing to notice the lack of distraction this family shared, and I could not help but wonder the last time I had experienced something similar.

Unless you have been living under a rock, you are constantly surrounded by distractions. These distractions could take the form of coworkers sending emails, texts from family members, social media messages from friends, or social media in general. You may also find yourself distracted by the sounds of kids playing outside, your neighbors upstairs, or down the hall. Distractions are everywhere! Take a moment to think about the last dinner you had out with friends. Were people texting at the table, or on their phones? Were you that person? What were the color of the walls, or was there art present? What did that food taste like, and what music was playing? The more technological stimuli around you, the less you are present in the moment.

Our world has changed tremendously over the last decade—heck, even in the last five years. There is an ever-growing number of things to pull attention away from whatever task you have at hand. Today, we have been led to believe that if we cannot do ten things at once, then we are not being productive. Why do we believe that if we cannot send an email while walking down the street sipping a latte and, at the same time, talking on the phone with a coworker to plan for an upcoming meeting, that we are somehow not keeping up? When did being busy become a badge of honor, and multi-tasking an Olympic event?

Have you thought about what is lost when you are busy keeping up? Many of us have forgotten how to be present in the moment. Did you taste that latte? Proofread the email? Forget to say good morning to your coworker? Are you truly connecting with what you are trying to accomplishment in the moment?

How do you feel when you are telling a story to someone

and they keep checking their phone? Have you ever been on a date with someone who texts others during dinner? How would that make you feel?

What would happen if you gave your mind, your energy, your spirit, and your emotion to the task at hand, or to the people you are engaging with in the moment? The next time you are with someone, truly be with them. Turn your phone off, and be engaged in conversation and fully present. Look into their eyes (not in a creepy way) to see if you can feel the energetic exchange between you and that person. For those who have social media as a part of their livelihood, decide you will capture the perfect shots, update the necessary mediums, and then put the phone away completely.

If you struggle with not being able to focus, remove the barriers that lead to distraction. Learn to set boundaries that allow you to be present in each and every moment. Teach your children to set these boundaries; what an amazing gift to give them. Express similar expectations to those you are spending time with, to significantly enhance your relationships.

A personal example you may be able to relate to is how my husband and I have learned to set expectations before launching into a conversation with one another. For the longest time, I would jump into a story right in the middle of him doing something on the computer or phone, and then be a little perturbed when the attention was not there. The same worked for him when he began telling me stories. Now when we want to have a conversation, we ask the other to let us know when they are free for their full attention (usually after completing whatever task was at hand), and then we would sit down and talk uninterrupted by anything around it.

Inspired Thoughts

MAGIC IN PRACTICE: LEARNING TO FOCUS

"Everything around you that you call life was made up by people that were no smarter than you. And you can change it, you can influence it. Once you learn that, you will never be the same again."
–Steve Jobs

No matter where you are, there are countless things that can be pulling your attention. Being able to accomplish what is most important to you is a matter of focusing your attention and working only on what you need to accomplish at that moment. A great mentor of mine once told me that focus is Following One Course Until Successful. How often does that happen?

Removing distractions and focusing on only one activity is a counterculture idea that will take some practice. To begin, carve out one hour each day to be your Power Hour. I do this every day. During my power hour, I intend to focus my attention on only one large task. I give myself the freedom to not do the task I have set out to do, but I cannot do anything else, either. For example, I set a power hour to focus on writing this book. As I sat down, I knew I did not have to write, but I could not check my email, watch a YouTube clip of my favorite reality talent show, check social media, clean out my desk, etc. Once all distractions and options were removed, it was much easier for me to choose to write.

Six Steps to a Successful Power Hour:

◆ ◆ ◆

Step 1. Block the time off on your calendar ahead of time. Let the appropriate people know this time is dedicated to your project, and that you are not to be disturbed. You may share the calendar with a significant other, put the time on your work calendar, or simply tell the people around you that this time is blocked off for you. Make sure you choose a time that you will be the most productive and consistent. If mornings tend to be filled with meetings, decide if you want to schedule your meetings around your Power Hour, or if another time of day would work better. When you choose your time, pick a time of day that you tend to have higher productivity levels. If late afternoons are filled with less energy and focus, then this is not a valuable time to choose. The purpose of this time is to move the needle and accomplish important tasks, so choose a time you will be your optimal self. If Power Hour does not speak to you, name it whatever will motivate you the most—Michelle's Meaningful Morning, Jenny's Get Stuff Done Hour, Chris's

Creative Time, etc. Make it your own.

Step 2: Make a brief list of what you intend to accomplish during your hour. Make it realistic, or you will become discouraged. Put the most important task at the very top, and make sure you do that before moving on to any other project. Look over the list and set the intention to finish your tasks and to do them well before you begin.

Step 3: Find a space conducive to completing the task at hand. Make sure you have the right kind of light, enough space to work freely, and all necessary supplies so you will not need to get up. Make sure you feel peaceful, happy, and successful in the space you are in. If you are working at your desk, make sure to clear off any unnecessary items so you can focus on the task at hand.

Step 4: **Make sure your body is in the right condition for optimal work.** Are you starving, or have you just eaten way too much? Neither are ideal conditions for getting things done. Make sure you have had water, and keep a full bottle nearby in case you get thirsty. Remove any reason why you would need to get up and pause your task.

Step 5: Scan your workspace and remove anything that will pull your attention. If the sight of your phone makes you want to check social media or message a friend, remove it from your sight. You can always set a timer right before you begin, to alert you when the hour is up. This way you have no excuse to need to see the time or have your phone nearby. If you are in a busy or noisy area, invest in some noise canceling headphones, or at the very least, a one-dollar pair of earplugs. Remember the rule that you do not have to do the items on your list, but you are NOT allowed to do anything off your list. This rule removes the temptation for negative self-talk if you are feeling unmotivated or do not accomplish your task. The freedom it gives you to not accomplish, increases productivity, but the ideal goal is to complete something important to you.

Step 6: Once you are finished with your hour, take a moment to celebrate all that you accomplished. When you do this, you train your body and mind to feel good about sitting down and working in these hours. A way to celebrate could be listening to your favorite song, standing up and dancing for a minute, high fiving someone nearby, or anything that will anchor that good feeling of accomplishing what you set out to accomplish. There are so many ways to document your success. Personally, I use a Passion PlannerTM to write down my goals and keep track of my progress. Celebrate the small successes just as much as the big ones, and you will get into a habit of fulfilling your commitments to yourself and your projects.

The more you insert the Power Hour practice into your life, the more you will be able to accomplish. You will achieve more control over your life, which will generate peace and contentment. Be gentle with yourself as you begin practicing this habit. If at first you are not able to carry out the tasks exactly as you want to, that is okay!

The first step in mastering anything is being a novice. No one ever decided to start playing piano and wrote a masterpiece that same day. Practice makes perfect, and committing to this habit daily will make it easier and easier. Remember, Albert Einstein, Winston Churchill, Marie Curie, and others, all had only twenty-four hours to work with as well. Look what they accomplished.

One last thing to note, if there is a project you keep putting off again and again, ask yourself if the project is important to you or to someone else. Work projects are one thing, but if you have personal projects that you are not completing, decide to either commit yourself to it and get it done, or take it off your list permanently.

Having items that remain on your list repeatedly begin to drain you energetically. It is acceptable to decide that it is no longer a priority and let it go. If at some point in your life it makes its way back in, you can recommit and go from there.

At the beginning of this section, I stated that how you do anything is how you do everything. I hope you have been able to incorporate the focusing strategies and the positivity practice into your life. Everything, from waking up in the morning, focusing on your internal and external dialogue and body language, to eradicating clutter and distractions from your life, leads to greater productivity and enhanced relationships.

Which one of these practices speaks to you the most? If something really resonates with you, take action now, and set aside time to make it happen. Remember, this book is only the guide, and true change is created when you decide to take action. If there is something you have read that you really do not want to try, ask yourself if doing it would bring you closer to what you want in life. Usually, what we resist most persists, and what we do not want to do most is the one thing that could make the biggest change of all.

Prioritize Your Life and Do What Creates More Joy

◆◆◆

"Holding on is believing that there is only a past; letting go is knowing that there is a future."
– Daphne Rose Kingma

I have encouraged you to eradicate distractions and focus your attention in a positive way. I know you have people vying for your attention and trying to get you to do what they want to do with you. There are family reunions, endless amounts of work, friends who want to go out to dinner, that reorganization of the closet that has been on your to-do list for the last six years, and all the other items that are constantly trying to get your time.

Everyone has a different capability of balancing these different activities. Maybe you can balance and juggle more than most, but at the end of the day, there is only one of you, and it is important to focus your attention on the people and activities that will bring the most joy into your life. It is not only people who are taking your time, but also specific activities that you spend your day doing.

It is important that you understand how you spend your

time, your attention, and your energy. There are only 24 hours in the day, seven days in a week, and 30ish days in a month. It is extremely important that you focus your energy and you spend your time doing activities that will grow your magic rather than steal it. This is how you will create the fulfillment you want and be able to show up as the best version of you, to those you care most about.

If you keep a calendar, whether it is on your mobile phone, your computer, or good old-fashioned pen and paper diary, please pull it out. Look at where you blocked off time for work, friends, and activities that you have planned. Calculate how much time you are setting aside for each group: friends, family, self, and work. Write what you have actually planned over the last month, not what you would like it to be.

List it here:

Activity	Hours Spent
Work	
Family	
Friends	
Self-improvement	
Health	
Other:	
Other:	

Do you see balance? Or is your schedule heavily weighted in one or two areas, while other areas are lacking? When you make a list of what's most important to you, does that align with the time you spend on your day in that area? Most of us tend to put ourselves last, while focusing heavily on our families and our jobs. We are going to turn our attention to creating greater balance in your life, by removing that which does not serve you.

Saying No Means a Whole Lot of Yes

◆ ◆ ◆

You can say no. Really, you can. Just watch, "Hey reader, send me a check for $10,000,000." Now, while you have the option to send a check, you also have the option to say no. Try it now, out loud, or in your head. For many of us, that is not an easy word to say.

We feel compelled to jump in and say yes to whatever is asked of us. At the core of many of us is this unrelenting people pleaser who wants to make everyone else's life easier, and does not want to be a villain by turning anything down. This is also true for those of you with FOMO (fear of missing out), so you say yes to everything, only to overextend yourself. This is how you end up with the extra project at work, teaching a class in the evenings, baking two hundred cupcakes for the bake sale at your child's school, or dinner plans six nights in a row. When you say no to that which no longer serves you, you have said yes to what you really want. Clear out the things that are not helping you achieve your goals.

Imagine you are in a buffet line, and behind each and every dish there is someone serving you food. You walk up to the first station, which is green beans. You are not really keen on green beans, but you do not want to be rude, so you take some. Next up is the mashed potatoes; you like these, so you say yes to these, too. Now you are at the sweet potato station, and even though you really do not like these, you say yes to a portion of these, too. Lastly, a big piece of turkey gets loaded onto your plate, causing your plate to nearly overflow. The last station is the pie station, which is your absolute favorite station. But you have no more room on your plate. So now you are saying no to the one item you were most excited to eat this day, because you said yes to items that you knew you did not want and will not truly enjoy.

This is your life! I am not suggesting that you ignore your responsibilities, spouses, or children, but for the extra events and time spent that does not serve your greater purpose, say NO THANK YOU. When you create more space in your life, you open yourself up to opportunities you never even thought about. So, take some time right now to write down what you can say "no thank you" to, and what that will do for you instead.

Here are some examples:

- No thank you to that pottery class that I used to love but now just do out of routine.
- What I get instead is a free night to catch up

on all the books I have been wanting to read.

- No thank you to my morning routine of watching videos on social media.
- What I get instead is time to do my morning energy practice, and slowly enjoy my morning tea in peace.

Remember, it is not about what you are giving up, it is about what you are getting instead. Here's an important note for you chronic yes-persons: just say NO to what you do not want to do, and check the excuses at the door. So often we are compelled to turn something down; in its place, we put a big fat excuse as to why we cannot do said activity, because we feel bad saying no. There are so many reasons why we do this: we do not want to be rude; we do not want to hurt their feelings; we are in the habit of making an excuse; we do not want them looking at us negatively; we do not want the guilt trip certain friends give when you say no; etc. It does not matter the reason why you have given excuses in the past; now is the time to let that go.

If you have people in your life who do not honor your time and energy, do you really want to keep trying to please them? As an introvert myself, I really need my alone time to recharge my batteries and feel mentally and physically strong. For my extroverted friends and family, this is really hard to understand. By making excuses, I am not giving those around me the opportunity to understand where I am coming from. It has also helped me better appreciate those in my life who not only honor but encourage my self-care routines, and respect my true feelings. So, the next time you would like to say no to something, simply say thank you for the invite but this time I am going to pass, and leave it at that. You have got this!

Dealing with Negativity

◆◆◆

Negativity is a state of mind, and if you do not like the state you are living in, it is time to move. I would like to think that most of my life has been roses and puppies, but that is pretty much no one's experience, and I am no different. Although I have harnessed positivity throughout most of my life by surrounding myself with good people, putting strong support systems in place, and experiencing genuine gratitude for every single day, there are still times when I get stuck, just like everyone else.

I had a negative experience over the past number of months that put everything I knew and believed into question. Every day felt like a challenge, and even with all of the tools and resources I have at my disposal, a very real cloud had descended over my day-to-day life. The reason I am sharing this with you is that I want you to know that you are not alone. There are moments in everyone's life where it feels like there is more going against you than going for you. I would like to show you how these are times of real opportunity for profound change.

Challenging people are put in your life for one reason, and

for one reason only: to help you grow as a person. When you recognize qualities within another that you like or dislike, these qualities will also live within you for a time. The traits we notice from people in our lives are simply a reflection of our own internal struggles in areas we can improve within ourselves. Now, this does not mean that you take on qualities you dislike. For instance, if you recognize extreme qualities of hate within another person, you will not necessarily adopt those qualities as well. Rather, when you recognize those qualities, the resistance you feel towards them is your struggle, and your struggle alone.

Since people are unique, the way you receive information is different than the way I receive information. The manner in which you process feedback is going to be different than how I process feedback. Understanding this concept is paramount when it comes to communicating with one another in a healthy, productive manner.

Some say that for someone to cause you suffering, it means that they have much suffering in their own life, which spills over into your life. Content, happy people would not speak so negatively towards another. In the end, hurt people, hurt people. It is not an excuse by any means, just a way of noticing that in every disagreement or discord there are two sides at play, and often we do not look at where the other person is. We are all dealing with our own issues. In my line of work, one of the number one tenants is, "Everyone is doing the best they can with the resources they have." The bottom line is that everyone has different resources, and together, we can help build up yours so that you can choose a different way to react when confronted with a demanding situation.

Have you ever flown off the handle for something you considered insignificant later? Of course, you have. Have you ever said something awful to someone you cared about because it felt so true in the moment, but later you regretted what you said? Sure, who hasn't?

Here is what happens when you are faced with a demanding situation. The area of your brain that controls your flight or fight response is activated. This part of your brain, the amygdala, has the job to keep you safe, and it thinks that it is helping you by turning on and causing specific physiological changes to protect you from danger. Here is the problem: normally, when this response happens, it is when you are stuck in traffic, having an argument with a loved one, or reading something upsetting. The brain, as smart as it is, is still operating similarly to when you were living in caves and had the possibility of coming face to face with a large predator.

A few years ago, I was at a Women in Travel conference, attending a lecture on emotional intelligence. Emotional intelligence is defined as the ability to manage other's emotions, as well as your own. In short, it is the ability to be aware of emotions, and manage them in a way that benefits external relationships. At this conference, there was a speaker who spoke about *amygdala hijacking.*[4]

It made so much sense suddenly! All those times when I

had an argument and said things I did not mean; all those times people said things to me that I did not think they really believed; those times when I was triggered by something, and my entire body seemed to be betraying me—even though I knew I was overreacting, at that time I did not have control over my emotions, so my body and my relationships were suffering the consequences.

Without getting too deep into the science of it all, when your body goes into this fight or flight mode, your brain overrides the thinking part of your brain, and opts for the quick response to emotion. It tells you that you need to act right now! I do not want you to think that because this happens, you have an excuse to behave badly. You are an evolved and enlightened human being, and you can begin to identify when you are in this mode. If you catch yourself suddenly in a very strong emotional negative state, where you feel not quite like yourself, chances are you are in the middle of an amygdala hijacking. The good news is, you do not have to fall victim to letting your fight or flight stage cause unwanted consequences.

How to Overcome Amygdala Hijacking

◆◆◆

Pre-Step: Though this will not help you once you have been triggered, I think it is important to mention. If there are situations that without fail trigger a negative response in you, stop to think if it is worth putting yourself into those situations. If you know that every time you open social media, your blood pressure races and you start commenting uncontrollably on everything you see, it may be time to take a break from social media. If there is a neighbor that rubs you the wrong way every time you see him, then avoid that neighbor. The best way to avoid amygdala hijacking is to avoid the triggers in the first place.

STOP AND RECOGNIZE: It has happened; you are in a situation where your brain goes into fight or flight mode, and it cannot be avoided. First step is to STOP. Before you say or do anything, stop yourself, and recognize that your brain has gone into fight or flight. Notice how your body feels in that moment, and be aware of the sensations going through you. You can also, in this moment, remind yourself of what you know you really want. If you are speaking to your spouse and an argument arises, stop; recognize the changes in your body and emotions, and remind yourself what you want out of the conversation. Doing this will help you focus on taking steps to come back to your rational mind.

BREATHE: When you go into amygdala hijacking, your body begins taking very shallow and short breaths to prepare itself in case it needs to make a run for it.

By breathing mindfully, you slow the production of adrenaline and cortisol running through the body. Focus on slowing breathing by breathing in for four seconds, and then breathing out for six seconds. Count in your head as you do this: breathing in 1-2-3-4, breathing out 1-2-3-4-5-6. When you allow your exhales to be longer than your inhales, you slow the body and heart rate, and lower blood pressure. This is also a great tool to use anytime you want to slow the body down, or even wind down before bed. While breathing, focus on your diaphragm expanding and contracting. Being present in your body allows your body to feel calmer, and allows yourself to be mindful of how your body feels.

MOVE: If you are in a situation where you can stand up and start walking, do it. If you are having a conversation with someone, ask him or her to walk with you. Moving the body helps regulate the reaction and will speed up the process of feeling yourself again. It also changes the physical dynamic of the conversation, because instead of standing on the opposing side of someone, you are walking side by side, which can change the dynamic of a conversation.

You have the control and tools to calm down during any situation. Imagine how different stressful situations can be if you take the time to use the tools to regain composure.

This is also an excellent activity to teach your children when they are going through adolescence and all that entails. I teach this to clients when I first start working with them, and it is amazing to see this light bulb go off in their head when they think about the disagreements they have with their significant others.

How often have you been trying to push your point across to someone who just simply seems to not want to budge an inch? Allow time for everyone to calm down, and once that has happened, go for that walk, and continue that conversation in a more peaceful environment. Remember what your intention was in the first place, and honor where you and the other person is in the moment. Not much is ever accomplished bullying one's way through. Collaboration will get you so much further, and often the highest intention of both parties is the same.

Inspired Thoughts

NATURE'S ALCHEMY: POWERFUL PROCESSES

"The Good Lord gave you a body that can stand most anything. It is your mind you have to convince."
– Vincent Lombardi

Our Emotional Bodies

◆◆◆

Being incredibly powerful, the mind can convince the body to do all manner of things perceived as impossible. Your mind will believe what you tell it, and then it will convince your body to do it. In other words, your thoughts become actions. So, what are you telling your body... your heart... your soul? Believe me, whether you are aware of it or not, you are telling yourself something.

What Are You Telling Your Mind?

◆◆◆

A person may say that they will only be happy when xyz comes along. I have news for that person: those things are now further from coming along. Being content is a state of mind and does not have anything to do with that new car, new wardrobe, or brand-new house. If luxury items were the be-all and end-all of happiness, there would not be any unhappy wealthy people out there, and there would not be any blissful families living in modest homes. We all know that both exist.

Imagine being in a movie theater watching a great film. Are there moments that you laugh, you cry, you cheer, or that you are excited? Of course, there are! And is that movie happening in real life? No, it is not. In the moments you are feeling those feelings, you are suspending where you currently are in life, and you are allowing yourself to feel the feelings that are being played out in front of you. You could have walked into the theater in a bad mood, and during the film, experienced a wide array of happy emotions. Or, often I walk into a theater feeling amazing, and a dramatic movie can have me crying my eyes out (this is why I tend to watch those films at home).

So, what is stopping you from feeling good feelings throughout the day? Nothing! A little imagination and focus, on the areas of your life that bring you joy now, is how you allow yourself to step into the magic. From there, the desires you feel, and the goals you have put out, get back on track towards you.

> Focus on something you have in your life that is going incredibly well. Focus on the gratitude you have for that. It does not need to be something huge; it can even be how comfortable you are in bed at night, the sound of the rain outside, or your favorite meal. How do you feel in your body? What is that feeling you have right in this moment? Really notice how this gratitude feels.
>
> Now focus on something that is not going so well right now. What do you wish you had more of? Now notice briefly how that feels. How does that feel in your body? That is the feeling that stops everything from coming your way.
>
> Now go back to the feeling you had first. That is when you are in your magic, and all you need is flowing your way. When you are in a state of gratitude, you are in the energy of allowing good things to come your way. When you focus on what you do or do not want, there is a stickiness that is created, which keeps what you desire from coming to fruition.

I have so many friends and family members who tell me that they are only focusing on what they want; yet what they want never comes their way. Here is an example: I recently asked a client what she wanted more of in her life.

She replied simply, "I want to be my ideal weight and feel

strong and healthy." She continued, "My energy is focused on the perfection of health and the feeling of a healthy body, yet it does not come."

Does this sound familiar? Is this something you have stated in the past or even in the present? I asked my client why she would like to be her ideal weight, and the response was a common one. She told me, "I hate how I look in my clothes; I never have enough energy; I cannot stand the way I feel most of the time!" She said this to me with more force and power than her statement of what she was wanting more of in her life.

Now, does this sound like someone who is focusing her thoughts, feelings, and actions on health or lack of health? You cannot fool energy. You can say the right words and pretend to think the right thoughts, but the true energy behind what you are saying and thinking is what is most important.

For my visual readers out there, imagine this: Every thought and feeling you emit has a frequency and vibration attached to it. For the sake of the example, let's say that the frequency of creating what you want is a vibrant gold, and the frequency of creating what you do not want is a deep red. When you think of your health, and there is a feeling of lack, frustration, or desperation, the frequency and energy you are emitting is dark red. This dark red frequency can be taking you further from what it is you desire.

If, when you think of your health, you are feeling grateful for where you are, focusing on how it will feel when you have perfect health, and expressing excitement for everything that will come when you have all you need, and feeling grateful for all you have now, then that vibrant gold frequency will be emitted. This frequency will connect to the people, places, and things that will make it a reality. You also begin to take back control of how your actions change your outcomes when you are in a state of deep gratitude and not at the effect of circumstances around you.

Have you ever noticed that when you have all you need of something, more of that seems to show up? When you have a wonderful job and are feeling great about it, suddenly, recruiters start showing up, and other phenomenal opportunities come knocking at your door. Conversely, when you need something, such as a new job, more money, or a better relationship, the opportunities seem few and far between. Much of this is an illusion, but when you are in the flow of positive energy, you are also more open to other possibilities, and are more likely to connect with people and be aware of more around you.

When you are stressed or not in a good space, you may get tunnel vision and shut down the possibilities around you. When you are in the flow of all you want to create, you are more open, and allow the treasures of the world to come to you. With this in mind, the next time you are focusing on what you want, ask yourself whether you are vibrating at a frequency that will bring what you want towards you, or one that will push it further away. If you are in a state where you know you are not creating what you want, stop, take a moment with a few deep breaths, and decide whether you want to change the frequency or not. If you do, clear your mind, and begin thinking of all the things you are grateful for in this life, especially when you think about your health.

Wouldn't It Be Fun If?

◆ ◆ ◆

Often, when we want to fix a situation, we begin to think about all the diverse ways we will change circumstances. The problem is, when you are in a negative state of thought, thinking more thoughts is most likely not going to help. It is times like these that you need to stop what you are doing and get out of your thought pattern. I am sure you have heard this one: "When you are thinking, you are stinking." That one always makes me laugh. As silly as it is, it tells you that when you are in negative thought, trying to think your way out of that thought may not help.

Here is a fun game you can play to get out of your head and back into your heart and be playful. This game can be played alone or with someone else. Here is how it goes:

Something happens that causes you to go down a negative thought path.

You catch it, realize you want to change the frequency, and decide to flip the script.

You look at the situation you are faced with, and

you ask yourself what would make that situation fun. You say out loud: "Wouldn't it be fun if….?" And fill in the blanks. You continue down that same path of questioning as you grow the dream bigger and bigger.

I really love this activity when I am with someone else because it becomes a game to see who can make it more fun. Now, it is important to note that this is not the time to begin ripping apart your dreams or contemplating whether or not what you are saying is possible. The purpose of this activity is to suspend your current reality and get into the feelings you have when you have whatever it is you want. When you do this, you open your mind to other possibilities, thereby allowing yourself to see options that were not available to you just moments before.

Here is an example:

- A woman is not satisfied with her current single-relationship status, and begins thinking of all the ways her dating life has gone wrong over the past few years.
- She realizes she is emitting energy that pushes her away from what she wants, and it does not make her feel great. She wants to play a game to change how she feels.
- She would like to feel light and joyful instead.
- She asks herself: "Wouldn't it be fun if…,"

and lets her imagination run wild!

- "Wouldn't it be fun if I got dressed up tonight and went out to meet friends for dinner?"
- Wouldn't it be fun if I felt great in my outfit, and I had a great hair day?"
- "Wouldn't it be fun if the food at the restaurant was amazing, and the company was excellent?"
- "Wouldn't it be fun if, during dinner, the table next to us started engaging in conversation?"
- "Wouldn't it be fun if we combined the two tables and had really fun and hilarious conversation?"
- "Wouldn't it be fun if we all went out to karaoke after dinner?"
- "Wouldn't it be fun if I really clicked with someone who was as terrible at singing as I am, but loved every minute of it?"
- Etc.

You can make the game as long or as short as you like. You can make large leaps to make your heart happy. The purpose of the game is to take you out of the thinking mode of where you are, and remind you of what is possible. When you are in question, you are opening yourself up to possibilities outside of what your brain allows you to think when you are in a negative headspace. The simplest way to start getting out of your own way is to simply ask, "What else is possible?" Even asking this one simple question reminds your unconscious that there is more available to you than you are currently thinking about. Statements can often create walls, while questions can often create bridges. Even if you are in a great mindset right now, take two minutes to play this game for fun, and notice how it changes the energy you feel in your body. Also notice when you play this game, your body reacts by standing taller and more confidently.

Hey Body, Can You Hear Me?

◆◆◆

I have always told my body that my triceps can handle around thirty-five pounds on the rope pull weight machine. That is the weight I have done for the past year, and it is automatic to set the machine at that weight. Once, when I was in Hong Kong, working out at my hotel, I set the rope pull machine to my usual thirty-five, and began doing the exercises. It felt a little bit harder, which I attributed to my lack of exercise since being on vacation.

After I finished on the machine, a tall, athletic man went up to the same machine and lowered the weight to thirty! With some effort, he began doing the exercises. I was baffled, so I verified with my husband that I normally do thirty-five pounds, and he agreed that I do. After further inspection, I realized that since we were in Asia, I had actually set the machine to thirty-five kilograms. That is seventy-seven pounds! My brain told my body that I could do thirty-five, and it did not even question the difficulty. If I had walked up to the machine and set it to seventy-seven pounds, there is no way I would have been able to do it, because that is what I would have been told by my brain.

If you want different results, all you must do is change your mind. How often do you tell yourself what you are capable of, because that is what you have always thought to be true? What else is possible?

How Worry Stops Your Magic

◆◆◆

"I have had a lot of worries in my life, most of which never happened." – Mark Twain

Mark Twain tells it like it is. How many times have you lain in bed, considering every possible dire outcome to a situation? On top of that, sometimes the situation is a mere possibility that has not come to fruition. Now, sometimes worry is the mind's way of indicating that action and problem-solving need to take place. This is healthy and necessary, when it leads to thoughtful action. At other times, worry can become an all-consuming beast that leads to unrelenting anxiety.

"Therefore, I tell you, do not worry about your life, what you will eat or drink; or about your body, what you will wear. Is not life more than food, and the body more than clothes? Look at the birds of the air; they do not sow or reap or store away in barns, and yet your heavenly Father feeds them. Are you not much more valuable than they? Can any one of you by worrying add a single hour to your life?"[5]

Most world religions share the idea that some aspects of suffering are connected to problems that have not occurred and, most likely, will not occur. Excessive worry is focusing the mind on something that could happen in the future but is not destined to happen. In fact, one could argue that it is the act of focusing on negative thoughts and worries that draws those very events to you. If you are insistent that something terrible will happen, you can unconsciously begin to manifest ways for it to happen, just so you can be right. Better than being right, why not choose to be happy?

There are also numerous mental and physical health issues that may arise due to worry. These stem from the inability to live in the present. Worries tend to draw you into the past as you reflect on past mistakes and what could have been. It also pulls you into the future as you fret over what might happen. Worry steals your present, but you can take it back.

How to Bring Yourself Back to the Present

◆ ◆ ◆

When you go into worry mode, you are either in the past or in the future. This state of worry is unhealthy for the body and can affect sleep since it will begin taking you down streams of thoughts of situations that most likely will not happen. A quick and easy exercise to bring yourself back to the present is a body scan and meditation.

Body Scan

◆◆◆

Lie down on your back and get comfortable.

Begin taking in deep breaths and allowing yourself to feel the air expand your lungs. To bring extra attention to this movement, place one hand on your heart and the other on your diaphragm so you can feel your body rising and falling with each breath. As you bring awareness to the breath, you begin to bring your focus back towards the present moment.

After you have taken a few minutes to bring awareness to your body, begin the scanning process by focusing on the top of your head. Slowly start scanning your attention down your body. Imagine what a photocopy machine looks like as it slowly scans down the paper. As you begin scanning down your body, notice any sensations you are feeling. Do you feel warmth? Do you feel cool air around you? What is it that you feel? Stay in the exercise, and if your mind should wander, that is okay; gently ask your attention to return to the scanning process.

If meditation or mindfulness exercise like this is new for you, that is okay. Just like anything else, it is all about routine and practice. Countless studies have demonstrated the positive effects of meditation and mindfulness practices, and we will discuss it further in part three. This is just one example of how it can benefit your wellbeing when you are in a state of worry. You can also do this exercise any time of day you want, to slow down and bring yourself to the present moment.

What you think, you attract. Do you want to attract what you are worrying about? Of course not; you want to allow ease and joy to flow your way. Therefore, you can choose to focus your attention on what you want to happen. See yourself living the life you want to live; remember that your unconscious mind is always eavesdropping on you.

Grow Your Magic

◆◆◆

A dynamic technique to combat worry is gratitude. You have heard a lot about gratitude throughout this book, and I cannot overemphasize the power it has to transform your life in a positive way. When you substitute gratitude for worry, you begin powerfully changing the course of your future towards a more joyful and fulfilled life. Some people call it a silver lining; others call it being grateful in all things. No matter what life throws at you, look for that which you can be grateful for. If nothing else, that contrast or friction is a terrific way to understand what you do want to have, do, and be. Be grateful in advance for that which you are working to create, and you will magnify your results, and shorten the time until it is given to you.

If this seems like a large task, choose a day that you will focus your energy on this. Changing the way you have always done things may seem daunting in the beginning, or maybe it will be a piece of cake. If you can commit one full day to making this change, you will begin changing your life. If a day does not feel realistic in the beginning, start with an hour. There is no reason not to begin. If you have never practiced gratitude, think of it this way: you have successfully practiced not being grateful in tough situations, and now you can successfully practice something new and different.

Take a day when you can be home, without commitments; write it down in your calendar, and then put notes all around your home where they will be visible. The notes should say, "Today, I will be grateful." When little worries or doubts begin to creep in, change them to a focus on gratitude.

This can be tricky because we tend to worry subconsciously. You may find yourself worrying about your financial situation, when you thought you were planning dinner. This change requires mindfulness and being present in each moment. It is not about perfection; it is about choosing a way that will bring you more peace and calm to your mind and body. When a worry arises, acknowledge it, then let it go. Imagine a leaf gently coming toward you. You wouldn't swat it away aggressively; you would simply waft it away. Watch it float away as you focus your thoughts on gratitude. It may help to make a list of things you are grateful for, to refer to throughout the day. Really take the time to get creative with this. It is easy to think of the items that everyone always turns to: shelter, food, etc. Dig a little deeper.

Once you have completed your gratitude day at home, do

it again and again. Gratitude over worry requires practice. As you begin to cultivate a strong practice of gratitude, you will begin to see how grateful your natural state chooses to be. Gratitude will spill over into every aspect of your life.

You never see young children worrying about what the future holds. They focus on the present, and live in the moment. Worry is a learned behavior, and it can also be an unlearned behavior, if you choose. Your health and the rest of your life starts with a single seed of gratitude that will grow as you nurture it.

Going with the Flow

◆◆◆

Many years ago, some colleagues of mine and I drove to Tennessee from Atlanta, to go white water rafting down the Ocoee River. Being my first time ever white-water rafting, and being a terrible swimmer, I was a bit nervous but eager to learn how I was going to make it safely from start to finish.

Because I am not the best of swimmers, I paid close attention to what our guide taught us. To my surprise, my guide told me to do the following: "Hold on tight, but not so tightly that every single bump will throw you around. Have some flexibility, and allow your body to move with the raft. If you are thrown from the boat, be calm, and make your way onto your back, with your legs floating at the top, facing downstream. Then, let the current take you."

Now, in my mind, my gut instinct was to swim like heck to get back to the safety of the boat, or swim like crazy to make it to the shore. But the more I thought about it, the more I realized my guide's advice made perfect sense. Just as a toy boat glides effortlessly downstream, so can we. The current of the river naturally flows one way, and it flows around obstacles easily. It is only when fighting the current or swimming upstream that the collision occurs.

Now, this is not advice to be complacent and just let life happen to you. But if you notice that you are continuing to strive against something, then you are out of tune with the natural rhythm of your magic. That resistance you are feeling is an indication that you are off-course. The good news is that you are learning the principles to bring you back on course, and your internal compass will constantly guide you back toward your flow, if you are willing to listen to it.

Healing Potion or Poison?

◆◆◆

We have spent a good deal of time learning about how mindfulness practice and other mindset activities can change the physical body, but there are factors that contribute to the health of your body. When it comes to eradicating worries and lowering stress levels, what you eat may help relieve tension and stress. Certain foods may help stabilize your emotional response to stress. Indeed, when you are stressed, your body releases anxiety hormones, adrenaline, and cortisol. These hormones are meant to be short term, but when consistently present in the body, they can start to take their toll. Certain foods can counteract the effects that adrenaline and cortisol have on your body. After all, you are what you eat.

There are countless studies and books written on the relationship between food and our hormones. I am not going to break down the ins and outs of what foods you can eat to heal your body—that is a massive book in itself—but I do want to help you understand the relationship between what you put in your mouth and the health of your body. Please see the resource section for recommendations on books to read on this topic.

Not All Food Is Created Equally

◆◆◆

"Let food be thy medicine and
medicine be thy food."
– Hippocrates

When I went to Rome, I thought I would gain a ton of weight because I was going to eat anything and everything I wanted. And I did. That is, I ate whatever I wanted: pizza, pasta, cannoli, and gelato, followed by cheese for breakfast. I expected to gain a few pounds, but when I returned home and got on the scale, I was surprised. I did not gain any weight; in fact, I lost it. How in the world was this possible?

The foods I ate while in Rome were mostly natural and unprocessed. I took a cooking class while there, and I was amazed by the richness of the ingredients we used. When

I cracked an egg into a volcano of flour, I was surprised to see this dark yellow/orange yolk landing in the flour. The spinach for the ravioli was so richly green, it was what I imagined eating pure energy would be like. I also only ate when I was hungry, instead of when I was bored, stressed, feeding emotions, or having unhealthy cravings, as I sometimes did back home. There was also the added benefit of leisurely dining, rather than eating food quickly, on the go, between meetings.

It has been well documented that food can either be healing or harming. The foods you choose on a daily basis will help you optimize your day, or potentially steal precious energy from what you want to accomplish. Our relationship with food is also a reflection of what we are going through emotionally. Oftentimes, when you reach for something unhealthy, there is a deeper reason than you might realize.

When I began my certification for health coaching, I was so overwhelmed by all of the conflicting information available: dairy is the best source of calcium and protein for you/dairy is the worst thing you can eat; sugar needs to be avoided at all costs/eat more fruit; you need meat as a protein source/vegetarians live the longest. The list goes on and on! These different concepts were not just varying; many of them directly contradict the others. One thing was for sure, I was going to need to dig deep and figure out what it all meant.

There are certain givens: deep green leafy vegetables are wonderful for your health, and donuts are not. Do you often choose a salad for lunch? According to Heather Mangieri, RDN, a spokesperson for the Academy of Nutrition and Dietetics, green leafy vegetables, like spinach, contain folate, which produces dopamine, a pleasure-inducing brain chemical, helping you keep calm.

If you were to begin researching foods for yourself, you would get more information than you could sort through in a lifetime. And depending on who was funding the studies, you would possibly get misleading information based on the results. There are, however, certain universals that most nutritionists can agree on. Here are 5 suggestions to start with, which will help you choose foods that are best for you:

Shop the perimeter of the grocery store. When you head to your local grocery store, the fresh foods are almost always located on the perimeter of the store. The processed and packaged foods are found in the middle. Shop the perimeter, and you will be eating more whole foods, meaning foods that have not been processed or changed forms. For example, potatoes will be found on the perimeter, and French fries will be in the middle.

Eat the rainbow. Have you ever noticed how many beautiful colors fruits and vegetables are? There is a reason why certain foods are certain colors, and they are linked to the benefits that particular food brings. Red fruits and vegetables, such as tomatoes and cherries, contain lycopene, which is a powerful antioxidant linked to heart health and reducing the risk of cancer. Blue and purple fruits and vegetables, such as blueberries, blackberries, and eggplants, contain the plant pigment anthocyanin, which is also a powerful antioxidant. Orange and yellow fruits, such as carrots, pumpkin, and apricots, contain beta-carotene, which is great for eye health and other health benefits. Green veggies and fruits, like kiwis and spinach, are the powerhouse of foods, and contain a range of phytochemicals that have strong anti-cancer properties. Dark leafy green vegetables are an excellent source of folate, as mentioned earlier. In order to maximize the vitamins and antioxidants you are eating, make sure that you eat the rainbow. Also notice if you are eating a lot of white foods, as these tend to be carbs, such as potatoes, rice, bread, and pastas. While they can be good sources of fiber, they do not have the depth of vitamins that fruits and vegetables do.

Skip the can, box, and bag, as much as possible. The closer you are to the original source of the food, the better. Once foods have been processed and put into packaging, they have lost some or all of their nutritious value. There are exceptions, of course, such as organic frozen fruits and vegetables, but as a rule, it is best to stick to the source.

Ditch foods you cannot pronounce. And I am not talking about quinoa, gnocchi, or açaí. When reading the list of ingredients on a package—and yes, it is very important that you read the ingredients—if there are words you have never heard of and cannot pronounce, they are most likely not great for you.

Eating time is simply time for eating. Now, here's a big one. How often do you sit down to a meal and do nothing other than eat, or maybe have a conversation? Due to the rising deadlines and the self-imposed need to multitask every single situation, more and more people are ditching the sit-down meal in lieu of eating on the go, or worse, eating at their desk at work. I get it; I was guilty of this for years. But here's what happens when you eat on the go or eat while distracted:

- You tend to eat more quickly, just to get it over with; but your body needs time to know it is satisfied, so you end up eating more calories than intended.
- You do not connect with your food or appreciate it. Enjoying your food can be an amazing experience. You do not need to be a foodie to enjoy a meal. When you take the time to slow down and really appreciate what you are eating, you begin to have a different and healthier relationship with the foods you are eating. And remember, since how you do anything is how you do everything, this mindfulness can carry over into other areas of your life.
- When it is time to eat, it is also an opportunity to take a much-needed break. When you take breaks and rest a bit, you can get back to the task at hand with more quality focus and energy. When you rob yourself of that break,

you are pushing yourself through activities throughout the day, instead of owning them.

- You settle for eating anything because you are in such a rush to get it over with. This is when you may opt for that hot dog stand, that vending machine sandwich, or anything else you can get your hands on quickly.

This last one is a big one. What is your routine when you eat? Do you eat while you are typing a report on your computer, talking on the phone, or while watching TV? Distracted eating is a slippery slope! Do you know how many chips you ate while chatting with your friend on the phone? How about the number of calories consumed while eating dinner in front of the computer or TV? It is not always just about what you eat, because your routine plays a crucial role as well.

Mindful eating does a number of things for you; it allows you to connect with the food you are eating. When you are more aware of the food you are eating, you will make healthier choices. Also, when you are mindfully eating, you tend to eat more slowly, noticing when you are full and need to stop eating.

Before I start working with a client who comes to me with health goals, I have them do a week-long journal. I do this for a number of reasons, but the biggest ones are so that I can see the relationship the client has with food, and so the client can start to bring into awareness the food choices she is making.

If you have been thinking about making some changes to

the way you eat, try keeping your own food journal for one week. Write down exactly what you ate and how much. Keep track of what the mood was when you ate that food. Maybe you will start to notice that you reach for ice cream when you get stressed out, or a piece of candy when you are celebrating. Remember, there is a relationship between the foods you eat and how you are feeling.

What time did you eat? If you are looking to be a healthier weight, but you eat dinner at 10pm at night, you are not optimizing your digestive system and giving it the time it needs to break down those foods before bed. And lastly, where did you eat this meal? Is there a relationship between where and how you eat, and your stress or calm levels?

Breakfast	Food	Mood	Time	Where
Lunch	Food	Mood	Time	Where
Dinner	Food	Mood	Time	Where
Snack	Food	Mood	Time	Where

Vegetable Broth (Health in a cup)

20 minutes prep
5 hours cook time
•Serves 4-6

•Purified water
•Garlic, lots and lots of garlic
•Fennel
•Onion
•Turmeric, bay leaf, rosemary, sage, thyme, pepper, salt, oregano
•Lemon
•Shiitake mushrooms
•Parsnips
•Celery
•Kale
•Ginger
•Carrots
•1 tablespoon coconut oil
•1/4 cup apple cider vinegar
•Any other veggies you love

I am including one of my favorite recipes for vegetable broth, which is packed with vitamins and minerals. Hopefully, it will serve as motivation as you tackle your homework of keeping a food journal for the week. At the end of the week, you may be surprised at the amount of food you ate, or the mindless calories you chose not to eat, since you were keeping this journal.

If you really want to better understand how the food you eat affects your mood, write down how you feel after each meal. Are you tired, lethargic, bloated, or foggy? Or did that meal give you more energy and vitality? How does the food you eat change your skin? Your skin is your largest organ, and if the foods you are eating do not agree with you, it will be written all over your face...literally. You will begin to see a pattern arise for the foods that add to your health and those that take away from it.

Mind over Body

◆ ◆ ◆

"You are allowed to be both a masterpiece and a work in progress, simultaneously." – Sophia Bush

There was a point in time when I did not even recognize myself in the mirror. I had not changed anything about the way that I was eating, drinking, or exercising, and I could not figure out what was going on. Why was the scale continuously rising? Though I am a big advocate for ditching the scale in lieu of paying attention to how I feel, the scale was telling me empirically that something was happening in my body. I was beginning to feel really tired and unmotivated, and nothing I owned fit anymore. I had been the exact same size since I was 15 years old, and this change felt like my world was turning upside down. I tried everything, and I do mean everything. I have a background in nutrition and, as mentioned, I am a certified yoga instructor. Additionally, I am surrounded by all the assets that one could need to create a healthy lifestyle.

Yet I was not managing my body weight. Nothing was changing; in fact, the scale was only rising, week after week, and day after day. It took a great deal out of me, and adversely affected my self-esteem. I entered a cycle of not being satisfied with how I looked and felt, which in turn created more of what I did not want.

I went to many doctors who said the exact same thing to me, "It is just your age; you are getting older, and it is easier to gain weight." No one would listen to me when I said gaining thirty pounds in a few months is not just age, and I knew something was happening in my body to create this change. And for the record, there are men and women in their eighties and beyond who are still in magnificent health, so your age does not need to be a defining factor in how healthy you are.

One day, I decided I was going to take back control of the negative chatter in my brain and reduce the stress in my life. It was a light bulb moment! The stress and the mental taxation caused my body to change even more drastically, and I was no closer to getting to the bottom of what was going on. This occurred at a point in my life when I wanted to be my absolute healthiest. I was getting married and wanted nothing more than to feel and look my best on that day. There is not a greater time in a woman's life that she desires to be in her best health and shape than when wearing her wedding dress.

We have discussed, many times throughout this book, how being at cause allows you to see opportunities and openings, when before, you may have only seen brick walls while being at effect. We have also talked about how what you think about, you bring about. If my unconscious mind was always eavesdropping on me, all it would hear was how frustrated and disgusted I was with myself and how I felt and looked. Getting my thinking in order allowed me to get back into the driver's seat and take action. I started to slowly practice gratitude for the health I did have, and for all of the resources I knew were out there to help me get back to my perfect blueprint of health and healing. Once I did this, pieces began to fall into place. A good friend told me about an incredible naturopathic doctor: Erica Matluck, ND, NP. Even though all other doctors I had seen had told me there was nothing wrong, and that I was simply getting older, Erica listened to me and really got to know what was happening in my body. She was the first ND I had been to, and quite honestly, it was the best experience I have had. After doing a series of tests, she got to the bottom of what was going on, and I began a course of treatment that put me back on track to becoming my healthiest self. I will be forever grateful for the time and care she spent with me. She truly listened to me and worked with me to find a solution.

At that point, I had options: I could have then used that diagnosis as an excuse and given up on myself, or I could have decided to act, though it would not always be easy, and make the necessary changes to get back to my optimal self. It all goes back to focusing on what you want, and letting go of what you do not want. Once I began giving gratitude for my body, for my health, and for all I had, other doors opened for me that helped me get back to where I wanted to be. If something is going on with your health right now, first know you are not alone. Also, know you are completely capable of loving yourself and your body, just as it is now working toward a healthier and more energetic you.

Fountain of Youth

◆ ◆ ◆

"There is a fountain of youth: it is your mind, your talents, the creativity you bring to your life and the lives of people you love. When you learn to tap this source, you will truly have defeated age."
– Sophia Loren

Why is it that human beings are the only animals that need to be told what to put in and on their bodies? Every other species in the world listens to their instincts and naturally chooses the foods that are best for their bodies. If we were to turn inward and focus on what our bodies tell us they need, we would make better choices for ourselves.

Instead, we often choose foods on a whim, or follow a craving that may not be in our best interest. And when it comes to what we choose to put on our bodies, it usually comes from advertisements, where the goal is to make money for the company, and not always to do what is best for the customer.

And some can argue that what you put on your body is

just as important as what you put in your body. Again, your skin is your largest organ, and it absorbs much of what you put on your skin. You would never actively choose to consume harmful chemicals, but you may not even think twice about putting that latest and greatest cream, promising to turn back the hands of time, onto your skin. There are many websites and apps out there that can help you understand the role of ingredients and how they may help or harm your body. A word of wisdom is to never take the words, all natural, clean, or healthy, at face value. Instead, do a little research.

If the goal is to have healthy and radiant skin—and really, who does not want that—then it is time to look at what you are eating, your stress levels, and what you are putting on your skin.

When it came to my own skin journey, no matter how hard I tried, my skin never looked like the advertisements. This was especially true when I ate a lot of sugar or dairy. Because I was aware of my skin's reaction to these foods, I was a little nervous about how my skin was going to react during seven days in Italy, where I fully intended to eat gelato and fresh mozzarella.

Much to my surprise, my skin glowed every day of that trip! While busy enjoying majestic Italy, I did not give it too much thought. A few months later, while in Europe for Christmas, my skin became so clear after only being there for twenty-four hours! Now I was taking notice. I had not changed my skin routine, so I wondered if it was the random products I had bought at the Copenhagen airport. I assumed this must be what had done the trick. However, after one day back in the United States, it all went back to how it was before my trip, even when using those same products.

I had forgotten all about how healthy my skin was during that time, until I went back to Europe for a good friend's wedding. All it took was one shower at the Munich airport, and my skin was so smooth, with no bumps or redness at all. After one shower! I realized it must be the water, in combination with the skin products I had previously purchased in Copenhagen. Since then, I have done a bit of research and learned the following:

- The water in Europe has much lower fluoride levels and chemicals.
- The products in Europe are free of harmful dyes and additives because they are banned. In the US, food dyes and synthetic products can be found in almost everything we ingest or put on our body. The skin is the largest organ, and what we put on our skin ends up in our system.
- My stress levels during vacation are much lower, and I am not producing the same stress induced hormones when I am not focusing on work and other possible stressors in life.
- The foods I eat in Europe do not cause the

> skin irritations that those same foods cause for me in the US. For example, in the US, I am allergic to eggs and soy. If I have either, my skin breaks out in a rash. In Europe and in Asia, I can consume both, with zero issues.

This is not to say that in other countries outside of the US, everyone has perfect and healthy skin. This is simply to bring to your attention that there may be factors outside your awareness that are contributing to how healthy, or not so healthy, your skin looks and feels.

Start to take notice of how certain products or foods affect your skin, and modify your eating habits and beauty routines accordingly. One thing is certain; it is always best to get to the root of the issue rather than seeking to simply mask the symptoms. If eating dairy causes your acne to flare, remove it from your diet; if certain foods cause skin irritation, choose other foods instead of treating the outbreaks with ointments or steroids. The body has a blueprint of health, and your skin and other organs are constantly working to balance the body. When you use products that dry up your acne, you are actively causing the body to try and balance the skin by producing more oil. Allow the body to be in a state where it is healing itself, because it is the ultimate machine of health when we let it be. Choose products that work with your body naturally, rather than trying to counteract it. It is all about finding harmony.

Move That Beautiful Body

◆ ◆ ◆

"When you dance, your purpose is not to get to a certain place on the floor. It is to enjoy each step along the way."
– Wayne Dyer

Have you heard of the perfect workout to lose those extra five pounds? Have countless exercise gurus told you that their method is THE method that will sculpt your body to perfection? It is all about moving quickly, running, vinyasa yoga, slow and steady movement, heavy weight, light weights—the advice is all over the shop! We are constantly being told that we will lose the weight and develop a rock-hard body if we simply follow the latest workout fad.

When we are taught about health, we often see photos of men and women in their 20s, running along the beach or sculpting themselves in the gym. After thinking a lot about the best way to stay in shape myself, I decided to ask my mom about when she last worked out. She responded that she had never worked out. I knew this was not true, because she takes dance classes multiple times per week, snowboards, and has walked the entire Camino de Santiago de Compostela (hundreds of miles!). When I mentioned this to her, she told me that her dance classes were not working out. She said, "That is just my body having fun; so is the rest!"

And there was the secret. When you find movement that brings your body joy, you will stick to it, and it won't be a chore; it will be fun. When you lose yourself to the pure enjoyment of an activity, it does not feel like work. You will have fun while bringing your body closer to optimal health. My great-grandmother was healthy and strong into her nineties because she carried her own groceries, gardened, cleaned the house, cooked meals for loved ones, and walked up and down her stairs daily.

Have you ever noticed that your body just starts moving when surrounded by friends and family at a wedding? When the music begins to play, you just cannot help but tap your toe and possibly start swaying your hips side to side. Or maybe you have a garden in your backyard, where you love spending time caring for the flowers, vegetables, and fruits. Digging around in the dirt, pulling weeds, and trimming trees all requires physical effort, but that is not what you are paying attention to because you are enjoying the process so much.

Let go of any guilt you have harbored because you have not done the latest must-do workout. Exercising does not have to feel like work, and you never need to set foot in a gym so long as you are moving your body daily. Choose activities that make sense for you. Find something that gives you joy, bliss, and excitement while you are moving your body. It is not about dedicating time to a long workout; it is about getting the movement you need to build your muscles and endurance, and keep your energy high. There are so many reasons to keep your body in great shape, which go well beyond how someone may look in their clothing.

By keeping your body strong, you are creating muscles to carry heavy grocery bags, your children, or maybe even your grandchildren. By building your endurance, you will enjoy those hikes in Hawaii, or even a friendly game of volleyball in the backyard. Not to mention that keeping a healthy body will keep many illnesses at bay. So, in the interest of keeping your body as healthy as possible, circle at least five of the activities below that you can add into your life for this week:

DANCE	CLEANING	GARDENING	HIKING
BIKING	ROLLERSKATING	WALKING	HULU HOOPING
YOGA	PILATES	KICKBOXING	WEIGHTLIFTING
MIMING	DOG WALKING	STAIR CLIMBING	WINDOW WASHING
VACCUMING	PLIOMETRICS	AEROBICS	RUNNING
JOGGING	SWIMMING	CROSS-COUNTRY SKIING	SNOWBOARDING
SKIING	WATER SKIING	WAKEBOARDING	CROSS-FIT
SPINNING	BOOTCAMP	REARRANGING FURNITURE	PLAYING WITH THE KIDS
DODGEBALL	PLAYING CATCH	BASEBALL	BASKETBALL
FOOTBALL	HOCKEY	FENCING	WATER POLO

If none of these speak to you, and there is something else you love to do to get the blood pumping, do it! Take a minute to write them down as a commitment to yourself that you are going to take action and make some changes. Once you get into this habit, you will notice you are parking farther from the grocery store, to carry those groceries to your car while working your biceps. You will begin mastering the art of the move your body playlist on your phone. The sky really is the limit.

Regardless of where you are today, take a moment to think about where you want your body to be a week from now, a month from now, and a year from now. What are all of the things in your control? Decide that you are going to take action to get your health to a place where you are thriving. If you are nowhere near where you want to be, be patient with yourself, and be kind to yourself. You did not get to where you are in a week, so it is reasonable to not expect it to be completely healed in a week. Visualize where you want to be a month from now, six months from now, and a year from now. Create a plan and take action! Find those who support you in your voyage, and remove the distractions that keep you from your goal. Be strong, my love; you can do this.

Inspired Thoughts

PART THREE -
SPIRIT

"And above all, watch with glittering eyes the whole world around you because the greatest secrets are always hidden in the most unlikely places. Those who don't believe in magic will never find it."
- Roald Dahl

You Are Stronger Than You Know

◆ ◆ ◆

In the summer of 2007, I moved to San Francisco. I was seeing a man there and decided to follow my heart and make the leap. This was no easy leap to make: I owned a home in the city where I was living; I had an excellent job; and my family lived nearby. Everything I knew was in that city, but in San Francisco, I did not know anyone; I had no family there, I had nowhere to live, and other than one neighborhood, I knew very little about the city.

Immediately, when I moved to the city, the relationship ended—it ended in a really bad way, and I was left without a home, in a new city, without anyone to lean on. I was driving around the city aimlessly, until I pulled over onto the side of the road and whipped out my little red Blackberry (this should tell you how long ago this was!). After scrolling through Craigslist on that tiny little archaic screen, I came across a listing for a studio apartment on the opposite end of town from where I was. I called the number, and sight unseen, I cut a check for the deposit and made the decision to keep moving forward, and there was no going back.

Since my belongings were in a moving truck making their way to San Francisco, I spent that first night in the city on the hardwood floor of a tiny studio, using nothing but my clothing as pillows and blankets. I was used to my three-bedroom house that felt like a home, and now, on the floor of this tiny studio, it was one of the lowest points in my life, and I did not know yet how everything was going to turn out. There were plenty of times where I thought about undoing all I had done, moving back to where I was, into the home I already owned, near my family and friends. On top of all of this, my house was on the market during one of the worst economic downturns, and I was paying rent and a mortgage on one salary. Even given all of this, there was a tiny whisper in my mind that kept telling me to persist, to be brave, to move forward, and to continue down this path I had created, and see it through.

I know you have been there. At some point in your life, you came into an incredibly difficult situation and were tested. You were not just tested; you were pushed to your limits, and maybe even past your limits. You were completely sure about something or someone; then, all of a sudden, everything changed, and you were forced to rely on nothing but your inner strength and courage to move forward.

The next morning, I woke up—if you could really call what was happening the night before, sleep—and decided to begin exploring my new city. There was no use sitting in my completely bare studio, so I got out and I began walking around without any destination in mind. After all, I was in a city I did not know at all, and this was before the advent of the iPhone, but I was not about to let anything stop me. I came across a giant hill—not a surprise in San Francisco—and instead of turning around, I chose to begin, step by step, walking up it. With each step, I was more and more determined to reach the top. There was something exciting about the unknown, about wondering how far the hill went up, and what would be on the other side.

When I finally reached the top, what I saw changed my feelings about where I was and what would happen next. As cheesy as it may sound, at the top of the hill, the beautiful Golden Gate Bridge revealed herself to me, and I felt deep in my heart that I was home. It is hard to imagine that I would move to a city before even seeing the most iconic landmark it had, but I had found it now, and it was a great reminder to me that everything would be okay. I cannot explain why I felt this way, but I did, and I never looked back.

Perhaps that boyfriend was brought into my life to change the course of where I was, along with who I was. I will get more into that later in this section. If you are in the middle of something difficult, and you feel a little unsure, remember that you still have yourself, and I will continue to show you why that is all you need to get through to the other side, where you will thrive.

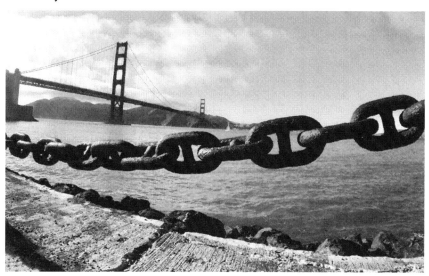

Inspired Thoughts

DEMYSTIFYING YOUR PATH: WHAT TRULY INSPIRES YOU?

"When we love, we always strive to become better than we are. When we strive to become better than we are, everything around us becomes better too."
– Paulo Coelho, The Alchemist

Years ago, when I was creating my business, I began doing what all new entrepreneurs do. I began thinking of color schemes, names for my company, my target audience, my offering, etc. I had been coaching part time for a few years, and it truly was the most fulfilling part of my professional life. I have learned a lot from my various careers over the years, but when it came to coaching, there was a specific kind of joy that brought out the best in me, and allowed me to bring out the best in others.

As I began setting up my full-time coaching practice, I was bombarded by advice from good friends, family, and strangers alike. For the most part, they all said the same thing—focus on what is going to be the most mainstream and commercial—so that I wouldn't starve. This made the most sense to them because it was the safest route, and the one that would not let me down, in their minds. "You should call your business, Business Accelerator, or Executive Coaching Inc., etc." I understood everyone's heart was in the right place, but this approach really never sat well with me.

If money and stability were all I was looking for, there were plenty of jobs that I could do that would bring that into my life. After all, what good is chasing a dream if it does not feel authentic to me in the end? My mind was a revolving door of thought, but my heart's desire was constant. Though coaching for sales and marketing has always been an area of strength for me, I never left a session as truly fulfilled as when I worked with someone breaking through a life barrier that had always been there. It was not until I went to Rome to spend a week with my mentor that everything came together.

Let me backtrack a bit. I was with a good friend and my husband, at a seminar focused on letting go of the doubter that lives inside of you, saying no to what no longer serves you, and developing a clear vision of my dream. I have always valued coaches and the art of coaching, but there was something different about the way this particular seminar approached everything.

The speaker was direct and loving at the same time, which really spoke to me. She mentioned she was moving to Rome to fulfill her lifelong dream of living in Italy. I turned to my husband and said, "If only there was a way I could work one-on-one with her, AND do it while she was living in Italy."

A short while later, she stood on stage and announced she was creating a once in a lifetime retreat for five women to join her in Italy. I looked at my husband with my eyes wide open. Then, he simply said, "Follow your heart." I am not even sure if he finished the word heart before I leapt out of my seat and signed up. There are a few moments in my life where my gut, heart, and mind were on the same page, and when I followed them, major positive changes happened. I had never gone anywhere with strangers, let alone to Europe, and I could not wait to see what could happen.

This is how I was able to spend a life-changing week in Italy with the fabulous Marcia Wieder. She has dedicated her entire life to helping people find their dreams and live them out. One day, at the beginning of the trip, she asked me, "What do you do?" This is a question that people ask one another all the time, though in that moment, it came unexpectedly. I quickly answered her in the way I had become accustomed.

"I help women break through their limiting beliefs and create the life they want. I help salespeople learn communication skills that allow them to serve their customers better. I help… etc."

She looked at me for a moment, and very calmly said, "I do not think so; what do you do?" In that moment, I could not understand what she was saying. My explanation of what I do was where I spent my time, and the results I had with my clients. For a moment, I even felt a little defensive, because I had unconsciously tied so much of who I was to what I did. She was looking for a different kind of answer. She wanted to know what made me different, unique, and special: what lit up my heart, what made my spirit soar, and when did my light shine brightest? There are plenty of coaches in this world who can very effectively get clients to the results I had mentioned above, but what did I really desire most for my clients?

"I want to inspire them to live the life they always dreamed of living, and teach them how to take back control of their life and make it happen," I finally said. Bingo; that was it. My mission is to inspire others to step out of their comfort zone and into their greatness. I aim to show people a life outside of the one they thought they were destined for, and into the magic of their own creation; to touch a part of their spirit by uncovering the passion, desire, and confidence that lies just under the surface of the negative beliefs and emotions they had accrued over the years. My goal is to re-introduce them to themselves—their true self—and let that person follow their dreams to the life they had always desired. Ultimately, you only live one life, and I want you to tap into your inspired magic. Be a magician, and create beautiful magic.

That brief time in Italy with Marcia and four other incredible women had more of a profound effect on me than years and years of searching for answers. In that magical place, I finally heard my inner voice telling me clearly what I had always heard faintly whispered inside. In an interview

Marcia gave recently, she spoke about how people are eager to get to the top of the mountain, just to find out they had climbed the wrong mountain. This has been me my entire life. I always took the safe road, and stayed loyal to the path that made sense and would be the most practical, but I was always searching for something else. I even spent years working in toxic situations, because I had made a commitment and thought I would have been a failure if I had given up. The truth is, the answers always existed inside of my heart and spirit, but I was allowing my head to steer the ship.

There will be many times in your life where your friends and family will want you to take the most practical path possible, and there is nothing wrong with that. It is really up to you to ask yourself if that is what makes you truly happy—the kind of happy that gets you jumping out of bed on Monday morning because you cannot wait to start the week; the kind of passion that only shows itself when you are on the path you were truly meant to be on. And here is the thing: when you are on the right path, creativity, abundance, and other things you desire flow to you.

Inspired Thoughts

SPIRIT AS ENERGY

"Passion is energy. Feel the power that comes from focusing on what excites you."
– Oprah Winfrey

Energy is neither created nor destroyed. I am sure you have heard this in your science classes once upon a time. Do not worry; there will not be a physics test of the end of this chapter. What this is essentially saying is that there is nothing new; there is only what has always been. It is up to you to transform it into an energy that serves you.

Energy is fascinating. We often think of energy as something in motion, yet it is so much more than that! Although many things on earth appear to be stationary and inanimate, all things have vibrations and create energy. If you had the ability to look at objects at a molecular level, you would see that the atoms and molecules are constantly in motion. This is why many naturopathic healers turn to crystals and essential oils to work with a person's energetic frequency.

Everything that is made of matter can be thought of as having or being energy, including money. If you think about money, it is truly just an energy exchange. That paper with the green ink or other colors is not really worth the amount printed on it. It is only given that value because that is the value we put on it. Back in the day, the currency may have been livestock, gold coins, or wheelbarrows of grain.

If I were to walk up to you today and hand you just a plain piece of paper, you would have no problem accepting it, but if I were to hand you a piece of currency, it would start to stir up emotions, either good or bad. Just as we discussed in part one, there is a certain shift in energy and mindset once we begin talking about a certain amount of money.

For some, a shift can happen relatively quickly, and for others, the amount needs to be much higher before discomfort sets in. And there are those who feel nothing but gratitude and levity, no matter what comes their way, and that, my dears, is my goal for you. If any negative thoughts come up with the thought of that, go back to section one, and work through those limiting decisions and beliefs you may still have hiding in your unconscious mind.

Rejecting abundance is nothing more than rejecting energy. It is not good or bad; it is simple energy you can choose to do what you want with. With more money, you could help more people; you could have greater access to resources, which would make it easier to live a healthy lifestyle; you could set up any number of foundations you choose; or you could simply choose to spend it in whatever way brings you true joy and fulfillment.

Money is not freedom. Freedom is freedom; yet for so many, there is a direct tie emotionally and mentally between having it and not having it. If this is you, look inside; and decide that this can change the relationship you have always had with abundance, and that having and being spiritual are not in opposition. Please do not misunderstand me. I am definitely not saying that people with money are more spiritual; they simply have the capacity to receive more into their lives, and you can too.

Inspired Thoughts

Where the Law of Attraction Falls Short

"Most people are thinking about what they do not want, and they're wondering why it shows up over and over again."
– John Assaraf

There is a major facet to the Law of Attraction that is rarely mentioned. I would like to share it with you, as it is incredibly important. When you hear coaches and motivational speakers talk about the Law of Attraction, they focus heavily on thoughts becoming things. Essentially, what you think about, you bring about. There is some truth to this: when you focus on what you want, you are more likely to obtain it. When you hear authors and speakers talk about the Law of Attraction, you hear them explaining that you need to focus on what it is you want, and pretend that you already have it now.

An example may be that you want a new car, so you take

the time to focus on exactly what car you want, and then visualize what it would feel like driving down the road in that new car. Imagine the wind blowing in your hair and your new driving gloves gripping the steering wheel. You have probably done a similar exercise, right?

When you are visualizing yourself driving around in your new car, there is a tiny voice in the background of your mind. That tiny voice inside your head may be riding alongside you, telling you that obtaining this car is completely possible and will happen; or, that tiny voice may be sitting on the sidelines, telling you that your dream car is impossible to attain. As you visualize what you want, this tiny voice is telling you that your first voice is an imposter. You can pretend all day and night that you will have something you are dreaming about, but if that tiny voice inside your head and heart is chattering in opposition, you are not going to move toward what you want, in a hurry.

Remember the seesaw from the playgrounds or parks of your childhood? You sat on one side of the seesaw and another child sat the other side. If you ever experienced this firsthand, you will remember that if you got on a seesaw with a child who was older or heavier than you, their side would tip straight into their favor, and you'd be stuck in the air with your legs dangling on the other side, not going anywhere anytime fast. So, to shift the weight, maybe you would ask another friend to join you on your side, and then everything would even out, and you would begin playing again, with the balance allowing you to maneuver how you wanted to.

Imagine your goals on a seesaw. If every energy and thought is in opposition, and there is nothing to balance your goals, they will remain stuck in the air, never touching down into your life. What provides counterbalance to your goals? After all, the Law of AttrACTION does not work without the word, ACTION.

Let's stay on the playground for a moment, and play a game of tug-o-war. The point of the game is to get the other team to cross over the line, so your side would pull with all their might in your direction, and the opposition would pull their hardest in their own direction.

When you focus on what you want, you begin pulling the rope in your direction. Imagine pretending that you have a million dollars; then the rope begins going your way, but almost as soon as you have the thought, that little voice of doubt inside your head begins chattering, telling you that you do not have a million dollars and will never have it. When this happens, an opponent is added to the opposing side. You may begin telling yourself over and over again that you cannot achieve this, while picturing yourself surrounded by golden coins, the kind that Uncle Scrooge used to swim around in during the cartoon, Duck TailsTM. And now, two more opponents are added to the opposition. And this cycle continues more and more, and perhaps you then start to focus on how far you feel from that goal; and by then, the opponent has won, and you may be left wondering where in the process you went wrong. You could be left feeling even further from your goal than when you began the visualization.

There are ways to gradually begin working on moving to the feeling of what you want. It is really all about getting on the energetic level of the life you want. Having money does not bring you happiness, but it may bring you the safety you want to feel in your housing situation, or the ability to experience the world through travel, or to take those courses you have been wanting to take.

Here is an exercise you can do to get into the feeling you want, without needing to jump all the way to the grand end goal. This does not mean you must give up on your dreams or lower your end goal. It simply means you need to focus on getting into a mindset and a feeling that will put you in a position to make it happen. Here is what happens when the opponent wins: you do not go after those big interviews, because you have that voice that says it is not possible; you do not accept that date with someone, because your energy is focused on the impossibility of finding that right someone for you. When your energy level matches the negative chatter in your brain, you are not in a space to be as aware of the possibilities around you, and you certainly won't move forward with the confidence I know you are capable of. Little do you know, when deep down your energy matches the vibration of a life you do not want, you can sabotage your own success, just to prove yourself right. When I hear friends passionately say with all of their heart that dating in the city is impossible, I notice they also choose situations to keep that story true. Do I think they choose it consciously?

I do not think so, and I sure hope not. But by doing so, they are able to continue telling the dating horror stories, and to show the world their assertion is correct. The same goes with how difficult it is to find a job, to get healthy, or to make more money, when all of it can come down to the desire and ability to give and receive energy.

The following exercise is meant to be a way to get out of the habit of going down the rabbit hole of negative chatter, and move towards what you want. When you say things like, "I'll never get that X," you stop yourself from taking action. There have been many who claim that jumping right to, "I can easily and effortlessly get X," is the best way to go. That may work for some, but for many, it actually creates this tiny voice in the mind that says, "Nope, that is not true!" Instead of jumping from one conclusion directly to another, try taking baby steps and feeling what that energy is like. Start slowly, and then move towards the mindset you would rather have. Here is an example:

"I am totally unqualified for that job I am applying for." Instead of trying to jump straight into, "I am totally qualified for that job," start with phrases you believe, without any resistance:

- I have been successful at jobs in the past.
- I have a strong work ethic.
- I love learning and growing in my career.
- There are people in this world who have been hired without all of the qualifications

necessary, and learned them.

- There are companies who want unique backgrounds.
- I am capable of trying new things.
- It would be fun to learn new skills and meet new people.
- I am willing to work hard to get to where I want to be.
- I am not the only person who feels unqualified at times.
- I have felt underqualified before, and have worked through it.
- I can bring to the table qualities this company does not even know they need.
- I really love working with individuals on meeting and exceeding goals.
- I have put myself out there in the past, and wonderful things have happened.
- I am more than the bullet points on a resume.
- Life is always working out for me and helping me get to the best situation for me.
- I'll never know unless I try.
- With every interview, I am developing new skills, and having fun developing these skills.
- It could be really fun to go for something new… etc.

If, at any point, you begin to feel resistance while speaking or writing any of the phrases, go back and change the phrase that gave you resistance. Resistance lives in the specifics, remember? When you feel resistance, bring yourself up higher in a vaguer area, and keep going. When you open up to possibilities in your mind and heart, you begin to see possibilities that were not there before; you begin to act, when before, you may have stopped yourself; and you move forward with more confidence. One of the very first lessons we learned in the book is that you have millions of bits of information coming towards you per second. When you are focusing towards your goal, your unconscious mind will be more aware of the bits of information that will help you move towards it; but when you are focusing on all of the reasons you cannot get that goal, your unconscious will pick out the bits of information that will prove you right in not getting it. For extra icing on the cake, move your body into a power pose. Do you remember when we discussed the superhero pose, earlier in the book? Move your body into this position when doing this exercise, for added oomph.

"Show me your friends, and I will show you your future."

This quote has been used for centuries, starting with Proverbs. Wise men have warned not to keep company with fools, and people in business have said you are the company you keep. No matter which way you slice it, the people you surround yourself with have a profound effect on your energy, your mindset, and your life.

Imagine that your personal space is your home. There are people you want to keep outside of your home; maybe they are messy, negative, or disruptive. They may be the people who come into your home and eat all of the food in your fridge, make a mess, and leave chaos in their wake. Even though this is always the pattern, we still let them in, because they show up, and we do not know how to say no.

Then there are the people that you invite into your living room; because, let's face it, that is pretty harmless, right? The living room has designated seating areas where you can assure your space bubble will not be invaded. Then there are those you allow into your kitchen; this may be a smaller area and a little more intimate. These are people you genuinely enjoy spending time with. Finally, there are those that you grant access to your bedroom. Now, those are the people you are normally the choosiest about. Keep in mind that this is simply a metaphor and not your dating life. You most likely spent hours upon hours talking the night away with your best friend during sleepovers as a child, but you wouldn't imagine bringing a bully into your room.

Think of the people you invited into your kitchen or your bedroom, from the exercise you just did. What is it that you enjoy about them? The people you choose to grant access to the most personal spaces of your life are likely people who exude a positive energy and make you feel good about yourself and others. They do this through positive body language, and they also use verbal language to affect positivity. They are most likely the people you can confide in, trust with your dreams, and speak freely without judgment. These are the people who support your goals and may even do what they can to help you achieve your dreams.

I realize that you cannot choose your parents, your siblings, or your children, but you can certainly be more conscious in the way that you interact with them. As for your friends and other people you have invited into your life, these are representations of what you believe, on a conscious or subconscious level, you are worthy of. These relationships will grow and change as you grow and change.

Are the people in your life vibrating at the same frequency you are? Do they celebrate your wins with you, and do they emulate the same values you do? Now is a critical time to really take a look around you and ask yourself, "Are the people I surround myself with cheering me on, or rooting for me to fail?"

It may sound harsh, but you all know that there are those "friends" out there. Often, it is not done at the conscious level, and their own doubts taint their judgment and behavior. Perhaps you made these friends during a time you were out to prove your theory right about why you could not have something. Regardless of your patterns and past, you have taken on this project and begun reading this book because there is something, or many things, you want to change in your circumstance right now.

Take a moment to think about the five people you choose to spend the most time with. Ask yourself the following questions: How do I feel after spending time with this person? Does this person genuinely want me to succeed? Does this person support my growth and change? Does this person allow me to be myself? Does this person bring out the best in me, and do I bring out the best in them?

If no is the answer to any of these questions, then it may be time to reevaluate how much time you are focusing on this person, and how much time you are spending in their company. Life is short—a cliché, yet true. Many entrepreneurs and coaches say that you are the sum of the five people you spend the most time with; if you want to grow and live a happier and healthier life, spend more time with those who want the same. I am not asking you to ditch your best friend since grade school, but if there is someone in your life that is a constant negative force, it may be time to evaluate what kind of relationship you want to have with them.

At the very least, give that person the opportunity to know where you are coming from, and ask them to join you on the journey. If they do not know where you are coming from and what you need, then you cannot automatically expect them to read your mind. If you have never asserted your needs, now is the perfect time to start. I will share a few ways you can cleanse your environment of negative or toxic energy.

For the next thirty days, practice incorporating positivity into your life and the lives of those around you. One of the biggest pieces of beginning a thirty-day positivity project is preparing everyone around you by setting expectations. I call it the Downer Detox. Let everyone you interact with know what you are doing in advance, so there is no surprise when you excuse yourself from unnecessarily negative conversations or gossip.

Gossip, by the way, is an energy drain and brings your vibration to a low point, far from what you want to create. People may find your sudden unwillingness to engage in gossip or negative talk to be a slight against them, if they do not understand what you are doing. Build your support system, and manage expectations in advance.

When friends, family, or coworkers come to you with their negativity or complaints—and yes, they will come—you will simply remind them that you are focusing on only the positive or productive, and gifting yourself with thirty days of no negativity, focusing on solutions rather than complaints.

This is not about pretending everything is 100% wonderful; it is about protecting your energy and focusing it on what you have control over. Since they will be familiar with your project, there will be no negativity or hurt feelings when your reminder is given. And remember, this is about what you need, and not about what anyone is doing wrong. You have chosen the people in your life, and they are a direct reflection of you. Once informed, they may become intrigued and wish to embark on a journey of positivity themselves. Imagine all the positive energy that could be launched into the world if everyone around you did this at the same time!

A few tips to get started:

- Actively seek out people who are on a similar mission to you. Join a meditation group, join friends for workout classes, or go to seminars on self-growth. If you have a lot of negative emotions to clear out, find a coach or mentor to work through them with you. Ask your friends if they know of anyone on a similar path as you; grow your network, and remember to give as much as you are asking for.
- Clear out any items that trigger negative emotions. I am not sure why we hold onto old photos of people who have hurt us, or old gifts that bring back negative memories.
- If the past comes calling, let it go to voicemail. You have nothing to say. If you want to move forward with your life, it is time to charge ahead and not look back. If you left someone or something behind, there is a good reason for it. You deserve strong, healthy, loving, supportive people around you. Let any BS go straight to voicemail, and do not return the call.

Apologize to those you may have wronged, and move forward. Apologizing, for most people, is a difficult task, because it has to start with admitting fault. No one is perfect, my darling, including you and me. Sometimes the strongest and most courageous thing a person can do is take responsibility, learn from their mistakes, and move forward in a new and better way.

Change your routine, and venture into unfamiliar places. We are creatures of habit, and we tend to go to the same places. So, if your favorite hangout always has the same people in it, try a new spot, with new energy. You will bring about different experiences, thoughts, and maybe even bouts of creativity. Find the places that bring you the most joy and passion. There are certain places in San Francisco where I get so inspired, I wish I had a guitar, some paints, and a journal at the same time. There is an office in San Francisco—an office, of all places—that always brings out so much creativity. The lights in there seem softer, the colors more vibrant, and words want to flow through me into poetry. I cannot explain it. Find that place for you, and let yourself be in that energy for a time.

Rely on yourself to complete this, and not for someone to make you happy or bring positivity into your life. This is about you loving yourself and allowing yourself to change your perception of the world, through different energy and thought.

And finally, have complete patience with yourself and others. No one is perfect. There will be days when this is easier than others. On those days, when things may feel like they are falling apart, instead of being hard on yourself, see the activities you have done throughout this book, and realize you have come a very long way. As mentioned at the very beginning of this book, everyone is doing the best they can, with the resources they have. This is my favorite presupposition of NLP, and it is also very helpful when interacting with anyone who is not in the same position as you, or when you are interacting with those who may have more resources than you (for now).

As you work through all of this, truly remember that YOU need to show up for yourself. You cannot rely on others to bring you joy or happiness—that power exists within you. You also need to show up for those who do support you and care about you. We are in this life together, but that does not mean you need to be the verbal punching bag for anyone, and you certainly do not need to be anyone's c onstant sounding board.

There will continue to be times when you are in a situation where you can get frazzled or booted out of your Zen space. That is okay; it is not about living the perfect life, but rather the best life you can create for yourself, your partner, and/or your family. Learning how to ground yourself will help make the hiccups in life less dramatic, and more of a tiny pebble in the road.

One of the most powerful ways to ground yourself is through the practice of meditation. Now, let's face it; there have likely been many, many people who have suggested meditation to you. Maybe you are already practicing it, or maybe it sounds like your worst nightmare. It does not change the fact that it is one way to help you move towards a happier, healthier life; so, let's explore.

Inspired Thoughts

THERE IS NOTHING WRONG WITH AN EMPTY CALDRON: MEDITATION AND SILENCE

"I think ninety-nine times and find nothing. I stop thinking, swim in silence, and the truth comes to me."
– Albert Einstein

Often, when you are looking to make changes, you focus on what you need to add into your life, what more you can do, and what action you need to take. While all of this is important, a good first step is to quiet the mind and center the body. Your thirty-day positivity project begins with learning to meditate. I know that I am not the first person to suggest meditation for a happier and healthier life. The benefits of meditation have been long documented. Some of the many benefits include:

- Reduces stress and anxiety
- Promotes emotional health and physical

health
- Improves concentration and focus
- Elevates mood
- Boosts serotonin
- Increases self-awareness
- Regulates body functions
- Improves sleep
- ...the list goes on and on.

One thing that is not always discussed when it comes to meditation is that it is the perfect time to stop the momentum of any negative chatter you have going on in your mind. If shifting your thoughts is not working in the moment, take that time to at least slow it down to a stop. Imagine a train going down the tracks in the wrong direction. Before you can completely switch the direction of the train, it is important to first slow it down until it has come to a complete stop; then it will be much easier to begin driving the train in the opposite direction. Since you have already practiced the body scan, in part two, you are on your way to becoming a meditation master.

Exercise

The first thing you will need to do is create a time and a space for meditation. Start slowly and be patient with yourself. Even one minute of focused breathing will bring about health benefits for your body and mind. The following exercise is a simple way to begin your meditation practice.

Whether you have never practiced meditation, or you are a pro, take two minutes to work through this exercise, and get ready for some Zen Magic. Start by clearing away a space so that you feel comfortable and calm. If you can clear away any clutter or distractions, that would be ideal. When you open your eyes after relaxing your body and mind, the first thing you see shouldn't be a pile of unfolded laundry or a pile of bills. Do what you can to create a space that will welcome you back with the same calm and ease you experienced while meditating.

Start by sitting comfortably in a chair, on the floor, or on your bed. Choose whichever makes you feel the most comfortable and relaxed. Shift your hips from side to side until you feel comfortable. Really take note of your body as you sit there. How do your legs feel below you? Are you sitting up straight, or is your back slumped over? It is important not to lie down during this time as you did during the body scan. Sitting is optimal for this exercise because it allows you to have balance between focus and relaxation. When you lie down, it becomes more passive, and easier to fall asleep.

After you have taken a moment to get comfortable

and settle your body, it is time to begin your breathing technique. The quickest way to slow your body and mind is to slow your breathing. Though there is an entire arm of Yoga dedicated to breathing (Pranayama), we will begin with simply breathing in for three seconds, 1…2…3…, and breathing out for four seconds 1…2…3…4…. When you breathe out longer than you breathe in, you slow the body and the mind. Take these breaths a few times until you get into a rhythm; there is no wrong way to do this part of the breathing exercise. Since we naturally breathe unconsciously, it may feel a bit labored at first to control your breathing. If it helps you to say in your mind, "In, 2, 3, and out, 2, 3, 4," it may help you keep the flow easier.

Now that you have the breathing part down, it is time to begin the relaxation process. Start by taking notice of your feet. Feel them against the ground if you are in a chair, or under you if you are cross-legged on the floor or on your bed. You do not need to shift your body or do anything; just begin paying attention to your feet. Now begin scanning up your body, slowly focusing your attention on actively relaxing each area as you come upon it. Slowly start scanning up your calves, then shins, knees, hips, and so on, until you reach the top of your head. As you slowly move past each section of your body, simply take note of that area—not good or bad—just notice it. Doing this simply introduces you to a new awareness of your body, gives you guidance to slow the chatter of your mind, and brings you back into your body with calmness and ease.

If there are thoughts that come into your head while doing this exercise, that is okay! There is no need to police your mind; that would be exhausting and impossible to keep up with. Simply allow your thoughts to float by you, like leaves floating down a babbling brook. During the scan, if you get stuck on one area, gently ask your mind to continue its path up the body. This exercise is meant to be light and relaxing. The more you practice, the easier it becomes. Just like anything else you have mastered in this life, you had to begin somewhere. And here is the good news: even one minute of mindful meditation is beneficial. If you need something more to focus on to connect your breath to the mindful scanning, simply think the words in as you are breathing in, and out as you are breathing out. It is enough focus to keep your mind engaged instead of wandering, and yet monotonous enough that it does not take away from your relaxation. Make sure you only say these words inside your mind, and not out loud, as that will stop your ability to take deep breaths.

There are also a number of guided meditation apps out

there to help you get started. Headspace and Calm are two of the more popular ones for your mobile phones and tablets. These allow you to listen to a voice or music that guides you through your meditation practice. Setting a daily alarm for when you are going to meditate will help you build a routine. Once you get into a habit of practicing meditation, you will not want to skip a day!

Now, here is a key step to do after your meditation session; it is a step that you cannot skip. Now that you have finished your first full meditation session, I want you to celebrate. Celebrate? Yes, C-E-L-E-B-R-A-T-E. It can be some people's natural reaction to start picking apart the process of whatever they just finished. Does this sound like you? Rather than even having a moment to begin doing something silly, like criticizing your amazing self, take a quick moment to celebrate in any way possible. If you are a self-critic, try this instead. Tell yourself two things you did well, one thing you can improve upon, and what action you will take next time to make the practice better for you.

You could celebrate by doing a little dance, singing a line from your favorite song, giving yourself a high five, throwing your arms in the air and yelling "YES," or anything that will make you feel good in that moment. When you create a healthy way to celebrate the small action steps you do to help yourself, you will begin to associate taking care of yourself, with mini wins. As you can tell by now, I am BIG on celebrations, and I hope, someday soon, you will begin to love them as much as I do.

You can do this small celebration in any area of your life if you want to change your mindset in a particular area. It is incredible how quickly you will cheer on your favorite sports team, your family, your friends, and even strangers sometimes, but you may be reluctant to celebrate yourself. Let that go, and begin seeing yourself as the amazing, wonderful, incredible, badass person you are!

Inspired Thoughts

BROOM FOR ONE: STAYING IN YOUR OWN LANE

"Action that is inspired from aligned thoughts is joyful action."
– Abraham Hicks

Now that I have shared all of these new tools to put you in the mindset to create and grow the areas of your life that matter most to you, you are ready to blossom. But what happens in those moments when your temperament is tested? What will you do or say when others oppose your new way of thinking? You will stay in your own lane.

I am sure you are wondering what I mean by staying in your lane. What I am suggesting is that you should focus on where you are heading by zeroing in on your goals and intentions. There will be moments when others will try to get into your lane, cut in front of you, or even drive in the opposite direction, directly towards you, and I want you to know that it will be okay.

Just like when you are driving down the road in your vehicle, you should be aware of your surroundings, but what matters most is focusing on where you are heading and what you want most out of life. Remember, your unconscious mind is always eavesdropping on you and, while your conscious mind is the goal setter, your unconscious mind is the goal getter.

Your chosen lane is full of possibility, hope, and wonder. You are heading towards ease, joy, and abundance by embracing innovative thinking, and by making thoughtful changes in behavior. The right path is not always the easiest way, but staying on the right path, and in your lane, will enable you to discover what you are made of, and learn how to triumph over doubts and missteps. At the beginning of this book, I told you that how you do anything is how you do everything. That was probably a pretty shocking statement to you at the time as you began to reconcile that your unconscious mind and limiting beliefs were impacting your life in pretty significant ways, which you had likely never considered. Now, I hope that statement fills you with hope and wonderful expectation.

You have many new skills under your belt now that you are aware and making changes to your mindset. Enjoy the freedom you have to create the life you have always dreamed of having. Take chances and be brave, for now is the time to own your destiny and move forward with courage and grace. I know you have in you everything you need to make your wildest dreams come true! This is only the beginning for you; there are so many more beautiful adventures ahead.

We are all chasing magic—that thing that cannot be seen, tasted, touched, or heard. It is only felt. What is it you are truly chasing? It is not a person or a career—it is that feeling of safety, security, and love. It is not a new car—it is that feeling of confidence and contentment.

In the end, what gives our lives meaning and fulfillment cannot be placed in your hands or even truly described accurately to another. Think of all of the millionaires who go to bed unsatisfied and unfulfilled, and all of those who have very little tangible assets, who live incredibly happy and fulfilled lives. It all comes down to mindset. The person who finds a five-dollar bill on the ground, and is thrilled by the happy surprise, may live a more joyful existence than the person who sits at home counting all their pennies, like Uncle Scrooge in his vault.

I work with clients to discover what it is they truly desire—what will bring them satisfaction—and how they can remove ALL of the self-limiting beliefs sabotaging success. Everyone is capable of stepping into their magic, and it starts with the mindset of knowing it is possible.

These are the last of my words to you in this book, but this is just the beginning of your journey to the life you have always wanted. You have everything inside of you to become an Inspired Magician and transform mundane Mondays into days filled with miracles, and conversations into collaborations that can move mountains. There is no dream too big or small, and there is no outcome that is impossible when you only believe that it can come to you.

Magic is when you find yourself in a less than ideal situation, and you use the power of your mind to change your circumstances by changing the vibration you are releasing into the world. Magic is when you see beauty when others cannot and will not. Magic is when you dig down deep inside and tap into the part of you that lives in harmony and balance. Magic is when you allow your true nature to shine. And when you tap into your magic and live from a place of possibility, anything can happen.

"Everybody has a calling. And your real job in life is to figure out as soon as possible what that is, who you were meant to be, and to begin to honor that in the best way possible for yourself."
– Oprah Winfrey

EPILOGUE

October 30, 2016 continued....

How does one describe magic? Is it even possible to do so? You know that feeling you get right before you kiss that special someone for the first time? Or as a child, when you would wear wool socks and rub them against the carpet with your friends, and then touch fingers for a shock? Right before the zap, there is a feeling of energy, of connection, anticipating a charge that is about to release and connect all at the same time. A sense of wonder, a sense of hope, a knowing that all is right and will always be all right because you are loved and you are loving. All of this, I feel at once, and I want it to last a lifetime. So, I ask myself now, how did I get here? Three years ago, at this very same time, I thought my happiness was over—I was unsatisfied with my job, had a boyfriend who just crushed my world, not enough money, too much stress, not enough time—and now I am here. How did I get here? That is precisely why I am writing this book, because I have been where you are. I have lived many of the experiences you have lived, and I have found the way to leave all that I did not want behind, and change my set of circumstances; and I am excited to show you how to change yours.

Be at cause, my Inspired Magicians. You may not like some of the things I lay out in the book; you may say that you are not at fault for your circumstances, that it all just happened to you, and there was nothing you could do. If you truly believed that, then you wouldn't have picked up this book, and you wouldn't be reading it now. You know deep down that you have attracted situations, people, and problems into your life, and you know that you want to change that NOW.

The sun has decided to show itself this morning. I did not think this place could get any more beautiful, but there it goes, showing there is always more to be discovered.

Where would you go if you could go anywhere? What do you do that fills up your heart? Who would you spend your time with if you could spend your time with anyone? What would you do with your life, if you could do anything?

When I turned twenty-six, I thought of going back to school and getting my MBA, but after doing some research and realizing it would take another three years to get it done, I felt like I was too old, and gave up that dream. When I was twenty-eight, I wanted to go to massage school because I was so fascinated by how the body worked, but it would have taken two years, and I was too old for that. When I turned thirty, I looked back at my life and realized that if I had just started my projects when I had thought of them, I would have accomplished those goals. You would think, at that time, I would have changed my tune and began acting on my dreams, but it took three more years, and meeting one very special woman, before that would happen.

There came a day when I decided that if there was something that I wanted to do, I was just going to do it. It all started with taking a look at my life and figuring out what was going to move the needle for me. So, ask yourself, on a scale of one to ten, where are you right now? What would move the needle a point for you?

Ah, now music is beginning to play below. It sounds like live music. The sun shining on my face, the sound of the breeze swirling around me, the fountain still singing its tune, and now an accordion plays somewhere nearby to signal the city that it is time to come alive—it is time to start the day; it is time to start living. It is simply time...

Epilogue

REFERENCES AND RESOURCES

[1, 2] "NLP Training with Dr. Matt." RSS, www.NLP.com/. Works Cited

[3] Nlpcoaching.com, www.nlpcoaching.com/tad-james-m-s-ph-d-transformational-leader/

[4] Goleman, Daniel. Emotional Intelligence: Why It Can Matter More than IQ. Bloomsbury, 2010. Amygdala Hijacking (this term was first coined by Daniel Goleman in 1996).

[5] The Holy Bible: New International Version Containing the Old Testament and the New Testament. Zondervan, 2009. New International Version, Matthew 6:25-27

[6] Adapted from the NLP's "Keys to Achievable Outcome." NLP Information, www.nlpinfo.com/keys-to-an-achievable-outcome/.

Resources

◆◆◆

"Experience Calm." Calm - Meditation Techniques for Sleep and Stress Reduction, www.calm.com/meditate.

"Meditation and Mindfulness Made Simple." Headspace, The Orange Dot, www.headspace.com/.

ABOUT THE AUTHOR

After working with coaches and mentors, and transforming her life in a powerful way, Michelle Hillier was inspired to become a Trainer and Master Practitioner of Neuro-Linguistic Programming and Hypnotherapy. As a trainer, she is equipped to help others learn to grow from life experiences, embrace new behaviors, and eliminate unfavorable attitudes. Michelle enjoys teaching women how to take charge of their own mental, physical, and emotional well-being. She realizes her love of empowering women through her Inspired Magic workshops, online courses and working with women on an individual basis.

Focusing on the mind-body connection, Michelle became

a certified yoga instructor through Yoga Alliance, and graduated from the Institute for Integrative Nutrition to become a health and wellness coach. Some of her favorite activities, outside of coaching, are traveling the world with her husband, exploring local outdoor restaurants, learning languages, writing, improving her photography skills, and reading. She currently lives in California.

Stay In Touch

◆◆◆

Website: www.inspiredmagic.com
Instagram: https://www.instagram.com/michelle.m.hillier/
Facebook: https://www.facebook.com/InspiredMagic/

Printed in Great Britain
by Amazon

55841939R00130